You Can't Eat Love

How Learning to *Love Yourself* Can Change Your Relationship with Food

Leslie Lindsey Davis

Resources by

Leslie Lindsey Davis

You Can't Eat Love Workbook

So, I said to myself... Journal

Fit and Food Journal

You Can't Eat Love Supplemental Workbook

Flowers: An Adult Coloring Book

(for a small fee, you can download the workbook www.youcanteatlove.com/workbook)

http://youcanteatlove.com/

Facebook group: You Can't Eat Love

Instagram: you_cant_eat_love

Find out how many calories your body needs per day.

Info.youcanteatlove.com

Books by the Pfishin' Sisters

The Untold Story of Noah's Wife

as made up by the Pfishin' Sisters

Reach out anytime, really
leslie@youcanteatlove.com

Dedication

Dedicated to:

my parents, who did the best they could.

my sisters, Kathy, Isa, and Allison, who threw lifelines to me just when I needed them most.

my brothers, Bill and Norman, who would come if I called.

my outlaws and all my nieces and nephews, so much shared laughter and memories.

my husband, Mike, who is wise enough to not stop me, even though he cannot understand half of my crazy dreams.

my three amazing sons, Philip, Jeffrey, and Matthew, who taught me that there is indeed a difference between boys and girls, and who love me even though they think I am crazy.

my amazing daughters-in-love, Carmen, Elizabeth, and Taylor, whose love for my boys is more than I could have wished for.

Joan Murray (Joan Murray Ministries), who believed I had a story to tell when I didn't even know the story.

With a prayer of thanks to...

God, who knew me before I was born.

Jesus, who kept me on the path.

The Holy Spirit, who gave me the words when I struggled to express myself.

For more information, email
leslie@youcanteatlove.com.
ISBN: 978-1-7362322-2-4
ASIN: B08RYC6Y8F

Table of Contents

SECTION I

WHY DIDN'T YOU TELL ME IN THE FIRST PLACE?

Whether you think you can or think you can't, you're right.

Henry Ford

CHAPTER 1

Pie Is Not Always Just Pie

I'm not in this world to live up to your expectations
and you're not in this world to live up to mine.
Bruce Lee

One Mother's Day, I decided to honor the memory of my mother by making several pies from our old, secret family recipes. The next morning, I carefully cut a slice of chocolate meringue pie and just as carefully put it on my plate. I thought about all the times I had carried a slice of this pie to a table. I remembered Willie Mae, Grandma, Grandad, Daddy, and mostly, my mom. I sat down at the table and slowly ate the slice of pie. I savored the richness of the chocolate and enjoyed the crunch of the crisp pie crust. I reflected on all the pies and times with family in the past as I felt the merengue melt in my mouth.

Then, at that moment, I really understood. Love is in the memories--the echoes of laughter and family moments. Love is in the doing. Love is NOT in the eating.

You can't eat love.

I had reached a point in my life where I hated to see reflections of myself. When I passed a window or a mirror, I would only look at my eyes. I would not allow my gaze to fall anywhere else. I would not even look at my shadows. I hated my reflection that much.

I was angry with myself for not caring enough to be healthier. But I was not willing to do anything to change. I was searching for a magic pill to fix it, to fix me. All the commercials that tried to sell me on their "proven" solutions had a mouse-sized disclaimer stating you had to follow a diet combined with exercise to get results. Even "proven" solutions were not a magic pill.

I would promise myself to not eat any chocolate. But when I got to the checkout lane in the grocery store, I would buy the 2- or 4-pack of Reese's Peanut Butter Cups and a Diet Coke. (**First lie I told myself:** Diet Coke cancels the empty calories in the Reese's Peanut Butter Cups.) If my lane didn't have any Reese's Peanut Butter Cups, I would buy a king-sized Hershey's bar with almonds, and sometimes, two. I would eat the chocolate candy before I got home and then hide the wrapper in the trash. Oh, and by the way, broken cookies and food from someone else's plate have calories too. (I know, I know – I didn't want to believe it either).

> A complete list of the Lies I Told Myself is in the workbook with space to add your own. An important part of this journey is the conversation you have with yourself. You are not alone; I am right here. For a small fee, you can get a pdf of the workbook, https://linktr.ee/youcanteatlove

Sometimes, I would go to the grocery store "to pick up a few items" and just happen to see the sugar cookies in the bakery section. You know the ones I'm talking about—the soft, perfectly round sugar cookies with the soft, colored icing piled high on top and a few sprinkles thrown in for good measure. I would decide we needed those as a snack at my house, so I would toss a package—usually the eighteen-count--in the basket.

I would load the groceries into the car, and of course, I always felt like I needed a "little smackerel." (Google things Winnie the Pooh says. 😊) A cookie would be the perfect thing. One cookie.

So, I would get the container out of the bag, set it on the front passenger seat, start the car, open the container, take out my one cookie, and begin driving. Three bites later, the cookie was gone, and its friends were calling me. They wanted to go too.

Of course, I couldn't stand listening to the rest of the cookies clamoring and calling my name. Before I knew it, I had eaten all the cookies and had only an empty container to share with my family. (In case you're wondering if I had to drive a long distance between my house and the grocery store, I didn't. The drive doesn't take more than fifteen minutes on a bad day with lots of traffic.)

Upon arriving home, I would hurriedly dust all the sprinkles off myself, swish some Diet Coke in my mouth to get the food coloring off my tongue and hide the empty container in one of the bags before unloading the groceries. (**Second lie I told myself:** Food eaten without anyone knowing you ate it does not have any calories.)

And I wondered why I couldn't stand to look at myself.

My family likes homemade cookies. I would mix up the dough and tell myself I wasn't going to eat any cookies. I would start scooping the dough onto the cookie sheet and then, occasionally, without my knowing it, a cookie would find its way into my mouth. Sometimes, I would make a recipe for 60 plus cookies, and only 30 would come out of the oven. I had no idea where the rest of them went. (We will not mention the number of times the dough had to chill, and no cookies got baked.) I needed to call the exterminator to take care of the rodent infestation because that was the only possible explanation for what happened to the rest of the cookies. (**Third lie I told myself:** Raw cookies don't have as many calories as baked cookies.)

Mysteriously, I had a similar problem with brownies. With cakes and pies, the pans were too small, so I had to do something with the excess. At my house, we have a septic system so you can't just pour random stuff down the sink. (**Fourth lie I told myself**. The pans were properly sized; I just didn't fill them properly. Also, we had a trash can.)

And I wondered why I hated seeing my shadow.

I remember having breakfast with my grandfather. I was about four or five years old. He was sharing wisdom about breakfast foods with me. I still remember him telling me bacon *must* be wiggly because the fat is the best part of the bacon. I took the advice to heart. I still like my bacon wiggly.

I took my grandfather's advice and applied it to other food. Brisket fat is the best and, according to "some research" (I wonder if the "some researchers" work in the same place as the "they say" people) brisket fat is good for you. Who am I to argue? Of course, that fact must apply to all meats with fat on them—steak, pork chops, and pork loin, just to name a few. I would eat almost all the fat from these foods—and believed no one would notice. I would even pull a brisket out before it was finished cooking "just to make sure it tasted ok," and then put it back in the oven to cook over. (That's where the rodents took a bite out of it. I should have kept the exterminator on speed dial). (**Fifth lie I told myself**. Fat has calories. Bites, including broken cookies and food from someone else's plate, have calories too. I know, I know. I didn't want to believe it either.)

And I wondered why my hips, knees, and feet hurt.

I struggled to gain control over what I ate. I struggled to gain control over how much I ate. I struggled to gain control of when I ate. I struggled with struggling. I just struggled.

I wanted a magic pill to fix whatever was broken in me. I wanted a magic pill for willpower because it was obvious to me that's what I lacked. I searched the web for where I could buy willpower. I will save you some time. You can't buy willpower anywhere. (**Sixth lie I told myself:** I was broken, and I just needed a pill to fix me.)

And I wondered why I didn't like myself.

So, I can hear you wondering how in the heck did I get from all of this to eating a pie and thinking I can't eat love. Well, I'm glad you asked. What I realized as I was eating the pie is this; I was trying to capture something I thought I didn't have. I thought I didn't have love growing up. I thought I was a failure in my parents' eyes. I thought I was not loved by my own children or by my husband. I *realized* the <u>only</u> love I was missing was <u>*my own*</u>.

I realized I had a *myself*-sized hole in my heart, and I was desperately trying to fill it with food. I was using the extra pounds to protect myself from being hurt by other people. I was using the extra pounds to insulate myself from the world because I believed I didn't deserve to be an active participant. I realized I was telling myself a lot of lies to justify not living my best life. Food was my "drug of choice." (I used food to numb my emotional pain.)

I turned on the lights and took an honest look at myself. This is what I call my lightbulb moment. (Thank you, Mr. Edison.)

Do you have a *myself*-sized hole in your heart?
Are you trying to eat love?

If you answered "yes" to either question, I invite you to join me on this journey. Together, we are going to discover our true, loveable selves. We are going to learn ***why*** we don't need to eat love. We are going to learn to fill the "*myself*"-sized hole in our hearts with self-love, not food. As you fill the hole, you will discover how incredible you are.

At the end of each chapter, you will find a link to all the sites/templates/books/downloads that are referenced in the book. For your convenience, there is also a QR code.

And yes, I am aware of some not so great grammar choices. I wanted this book to sound as if we are simply two very good friends enjoying a conversation. I wanted to stay true to the way I speak.

CHAPTER 2

You Can Begin Again with a Trip

I have always loved the first day of school better than the last. Firsts are best because they are beginnings.

Jenny Han

To begin, begin.

Peter Nixio Zarlenga

So, start packing. We are going on a trip! Get out your favorite suitcase. Mine is a zebra print with pink trim—quite easy to spot in the airport. Show me your favorite suitcase; you can post a picture on our closed You Can't Eat Love Facebook page.

Oh, and toss in a few pens and a highlighter. As we travel, we will be putting more things in our suitcases. At the end of each chapter, I will let you know what to add and remind you what is already in there.

Since we are going to get to know each other very well, I wanted to explain a few things before we start on our journey. I have tried and failed (we will talk more about failing later) more diets than I can count. You may have too. I want to help you begin to love yourself, and most importantly, believe in yourself so you can change your relationship with food—and get off the diet merry-go-round.

In this book, I am going to show you how to change shaming and blaming thoughts into loving and kind thoughts. I am going to show you how to become your very best friend in the whole wide world. I am going to show you how to fill the *"myself"*-sized hole in your heart with love, one shovelful at a time. You will *never* be doing this work alone.

I hit a place in my life where I had to make some decisions. Either I would keep going down the road I was on and ***not*** live my best life, or I would make some drastic changes. *I chose to make some changes*. I literally drove a stake in the ground and declared the old Leslie was gone and Leslie 2.0 was beginning. If every brand, car, food, and software, could be new and improved, why not me? Leslie 2.0 was ready to try something else.

Changing was *not* easy, but I was and am worth it. I did follow the Weight Watchers food plan, but that was not the hard part. The hard part was doing the hard work: discovering the real me, taking care of the very scared, little girl hiding behind all the weight, learning to handle the critical parent locked in my head, and believing I deserved love. As I learned I did deserve love, the weight came off easier and easier. I shed fear, rejection, self-hate, and self-loathing. I lost almost one hundred pounds and discovered I *could* love myself.

After reading my book, you will be able to speak kindly to yourself. You will know how to create plans of action for different food situations and celebrations that revolve around food. You will know how to practice for these occasions. You will know how to ask for *and get* what you need. After reading my book, you will be well on your way to filling the *myself*-sized hole in your heart. And you will learn you are never alone.

I invite you to visit the *You Can't Eat Love* website to see lots of before, after, and now photos. Two years after reaching the weight I knew I could live with, I decided to fall in love with deadlifting. I have added incredible muscle and strength because of this new part of my journey. Please join our closed Facebook group so the community can share with you and support you on your journey. We are all about cheering each other on. No shaming or shoulding allowed!

After you have read *You Can't Eat Love*, I promise you will never look at another trip the same way again. You will never look at an oxygen mask the same way again. And you will remove the word diet from your vocabulary. I promise you will discover your very best friend in the whole wide world.

Why pass up the chance to live the very best life you deserve now? Life is too short to not speak to yourself with kindness and caring. Life is too short for shaming and shoulding.

Grab your suitcase. Make sure you have your workbook, journal, pens, and highlighters. Don't worry; we will pick up the other things we need along the way. If you would like, post a photo of your suitcase on Facebook, so we can let you know how excited we are to have you on this journey with us. We have plenty of room in the car for you. We will even let you have a turn choosing the tunes.

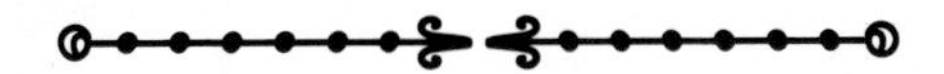

What's in your suitcase?

- Snap a photo – post it to the You Can't Eat Love Facebook page
- Join the private You Can't Eat Love Facebook group
- You Can't Eat Love Workbook (www.youcanteatlove.com/workbook)
- So, I said to myself... Journal (you can get it here https://youcanteatlove.com/you-cant-eat-love-series)
- Pens (I like using crazy colored pens, but any kind of pens will work.)

- Highlighters
- Paper (You never know when you will want to write something down.)

Life Hacks

- This journey is about choosing you. Decide on a time of day you can spend quality time with you. Either create a reminder on your phone or write it on your calendar. If you decide the best time is early in the morning while the house is quiet, commit to setting your alarm to get up just ten minutes early. Say to yourself – ***I'm choosing me***. Write it down.

- Start noticing how you are speaking to yourself. Notice how other people are speaking to you. Go to www.youcanteatlove.com/journal to download sample pages so you can begin having conversations with yourself.

- Name the inner voices. I call the ones that don't speak nicely to you monsters, the critics, and the hamsters on wheels. Feel free to substitute whatever you call them but do name them. Also, traveling on this journey are two four-year-old children (a brat and a scared child), two parents (one critical and one kind), and your very best friend in the whole wide world.

- Take hold of a life jacket. Sometimes I will toss you one. You can toss one to me too. Sometimes we need a life jacket because we are tired of swimming and just need to float a bit, so we can rest and get ready to swim again. It is ok to grab a life jacket and hold on. You don't have to give it back. You can keep it for the next time you need to rest. Trust me. There will be a next time.

- I share lots of expressions and sayings. Please feel free to use them and modify them. Let me know what does and doesn't work for you.

- I tell a lot of stories, and I hope you learn a little something from them. I do want to hear your stories. I can learn a lot from you too. Remember, we are going to be traveling together. It will not be much fun if I am doing all the talking. You can tell me about ***your*** stories on Facebook or leslie@youcanteatlove.com.

- At the end of each chapter, I will share tips and tricks (Life Hacks) I discovered along the way.

- I will include links to all types of information, questionnaires, and resources. A lot of the life hacks information is included in the workbook. For a small fee, you can order a pdf at www.youcanteatlove.com/workbook. You can also find information to order the workbook on the website https://youcanteatlove.com/you-cant-eat-love-series

- The amazing Jackie will also be sharing how to add activity and exercise into your life at your pace. Jacqueline "Jackie" Lewandowski is a licensed Certified Personal Trainer with over 15 years of experience. We all need a Jackie in our lives.

- This is not a diet. You are changing your lifestyle. So, remove any thoughts of a diet from your mind.

Remove the word diet from your vocabulary.

- At the end of each chapter, I will have a link and a QR code that will list all the websites referenced.

Jackie says

- Start slow
- Meet you where you are
- Drink lots of water

Weblinks

https://linktr.ee/youcanteatlove

CHAPTER 3

Pack Your Suitcase

A journey of a thousand miles begins with a single step.
Attributed to Lau-Tzu

I love to travel, but I don't like packing my suitcase. Why not? Because I know I have to unpack it when I get home. Unpacking involves washing all the dirty laundry, putting my things back in place, and figuring out where to put all the treasures I picked up on the trip. I think about all of that while I am packing.

But when I start thinking about where I am going, I forget about all the things I must do when I get back. I make sure I have the right clothes, the right shoes, a hat, pj's, a toothbrush, and all that stuff. I start to get excited about leaving and focus on what's next so I can get on my way.

Please hang in here with me. We already have our suitcases out, and we have packed a few things. Now, we are going to pack our oxygen masks. I can already hear your questions.

"Oxygen mask? Why do I need an oxygen mask?"

Have you ever flown on an airplane? Do you remember the flight instructions? They tell you if there is trouble on the airplane, the first thing you must do is put on your own oxygen mask. You must do this before you do anything else.

Do you watch any medical shows with ambulances and emergencies? What is one of the first things the medical staff does? They put an oxygen mask on the patient. Then they start trying to figure out what is going on.

So, why do you need your oxygen mask for this trip? Because you will soon begin to realize how many times you are helping someone else put on their oxygen mask and leaving yourself gasping for air, or worse. Remember that *myself*-sized hole in your heart you are trying to fill? Trust me, you need an oxygen mask. Put it in the suitcase. We will talk about oxygen masks some more as we travel (such as when we need something to talk about to keep our minds off the boring parts of the trip).

Now, this is the most important part of your trip. Make sure you are taking this trip for the right reason and that you get on the right road. You don't want to travel all that way only to arrive somewhere and wonder what the heck you are doing there.

Before you zip up your suitcase, get out a pen, your workbook, and maybe some extra paper. You may even want to grab your favorite beverage and a stack of tissues. Find a quiet place where you can sit down by yourself with these things.

I want you to be honest with yourself. Super "deep down to your toes" honest. No one else is going to see what you write unless you share it with them.

I want you to tell yourself ***WHY*** you want to lose weight. ***WHY*** is not the goal; it is the reason to keep moving forward when all you want to do is stop and give up. This is your specific ***WHY*** and not someone else's. Your ***WHY*** is not an event or a number.

I challenge you to be what I call "tears running down your face" honest with yourself. Keep writing all the thoughts, dreams, fears, and beliefs that come to mind until you are absolutely and totally drained. Remember the stack of tissues? Use it; you can always pack more.

I'm going to ask you a few questions (these questions are also in the workbook) to help you dig down deep and discover *your* ***WHY***. Fear not. I will still be here when you finish pouring out your heart to yourself.

Finding you so you can discover your why

1. What excites you? Think about things you like to do and places you like to go.
   ____
   ____
   ____
   ____

2. On a scale of 1-5 (1 is extremely unhappy and 5 is extremely happy), rate how you feel about the following areas of your life:
   Health ____ Friends ____ Family ____ Recreation (Fun) ____ Personal Growth ____

3. Now write *why* you gave each of those areas the rating you did. Be honest. Remember, no one else is going to see this unless you decide to share it with them.
   Health____
   ____
   ____
   ____
   Friends_______________________________________
   ____
   ____
   ____
   Family____
   ____
   ____
   Recreation(Fun)______________________________

PersonalGrowth

What do you *believe* you cannot do? (Yes, losing weight can be one of those things.)

4. What would your life look like if you believed you *could* do those things? (If you need to, channel your thoughts toward The *Little Engine That Could* by Watty Piper.)

5. What was your relationship with food ten years ago?

6. What is your relationship with food today? What changed? Why do you think it changed?

7. What are your fears and why? List as many fears as you can think of. Failure and success can both be fears. I am afraid of

____

____

____

____

____

because (Keep going! You've got this!)

____

____

____

____

____

____

____

____

8. Pick one of your fears and think about how it would feel to act against just that one fear. What would that look like?

____

____

____

____

____

____

9. List the challenges you have had over the past year.

____

____

____

____

10. What did you learn about yourself from these challenges?

____

____

____

____

11. Following is my long-time mantra: I don't want to be 80 years old, sitting on my front porch in my rocker and saying I wish I would have...
    Now it is your turn to fill in the blank...

    ____

    ____

    ____

    ____

    ____

    ____

    ____

    ____

12. Fill in these blanks: My name is

    ______________________________.

    I am (not a job title or diet failure)

    ____

    ____

    In the past, I have (had what kind of relationship/belief system about food)

    ____

    ____,

    but now I am ready to (describe what kind of relationship you want with yourself, not food).

    ____

    ____

    This is important to me because (nothing to do with your weight, another person, or an event).

    ____

    ____

    ____

    WHY I want to reclaim myself matters. I am important to me.

You can go to http://youcanteatlove.com/mywhy to see the interview about *my* ***WHY.***

Why

You are probably going to wonder why I did not tell you this next part first. I wanted you to dig down deep and really start connecting with the *you* that is running around inside your head. You are going to get to know that person very well, and if I cluttered up your head with *me*, we would never get to *you*.

So, now, back to our trip.

For quite a few years, I thought *why* the same thing as a goal was. I was fairly good at coming up with goals. After all, isn't that what New Year's Resolutions are? What I was terrible at was reaching the goals I so carefully planned out. I just did not understand how come I either quickly forgot the goals or got tired of chasing them. After all, I clearly understood the framework of a good goal—you know that whole S.M.A.R.T. thing. I could do that all day long, with one hand tied behind my back. What they (there are those "they" people again) don't teach you is that while it is great to have these fancy S.M.A.R.T. goals, they are not worth the paper they are printed on *if* you are not crystal clear on ***WHY.***

Sometimes, when we are questioned about our ***WHY,*** it is easier to just answer "Because" and walk away. ***WHY*** can be hard to explain to someone who has never been desperate. Your personal ***WHY*** can be plain hard to explain to anyone. And that is ok. It is *your* ***WHY.***

WHY is what helps us figure out ***how***. Friedrich Nietzsche said, "If we have our own why in life, we shall get along with almost any how." ***WHY*** is what gets you up in the morning. ***WHY*** is what keeps you going when you are tired of running into obstacles. Think of your ***WHY*** as your north star—your lighthouse that keeps you from smashing into the rocks. *Your* ***WHY*** is also what gets you off the rocks if you do smash into them.

> You can download a beautiful copy of this quote and add your own why to it https://bit.ly/33Bu1AN

Go ahead and pack your ***WHY*** where you can quickly get to it—right next to your oxygen mask is a good place.

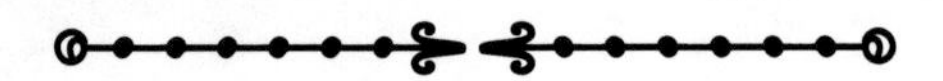

What's in your suitcase?

- Oxygen mask
- WHY
- Friedrich Nietzche quote
- Photo of you
- Index cards
- Stake
- Hammer
- http://youcanteatlove.com
- Snap a photo – post it to the Facebook page
- Join the private You Can't Eat Love Facebook group
- Workbook
- *So, I said to myself...* Journal
- Pens
- Highlighters

Life Hacks

- Each month, as I plan for the month ahead, I write this same note to myself on my planner: "I'm MY #1 priority". This is a code I have come up with to gently remind myself of my WHY without sharing it with anyone else. You can borrow my note or come up with a few of your own.

- I copied my WHY onto several index cards and keep them in strategic places (like my planner, my inspirational reading books) so I can remind myself why I'm on this journey. I don't leave it out for the general public to see.
- After you create your WHY, find a photo of yourself that makes you smile at the memory of when the photo was taken. Make copies of that photo and put them with your copies of your WHY. I want you to recall the feeling the memory reminds you of. Drop a copy in your suitcase while you're at it!
- On the website, there is a supplemental workbook available if you are still struggling to get clear on your WHY. You can also reach out to me for a chat and I will help you get clear.

Jackie says

- Find your WHY
- Take progress pictures

Weblinks

https://linktr.ee/youcanteatlove

CHAPTER 4

It's Not About the Destination

It's a mistake to look too far ahead on the chain of destiny.
We can only handle one link at a time.

Winston Churchill

I want you to think back to the longest trip you have ever been on. To me, the easiest way to think about this is traveling by plane. If you have never flown, that's ok, just think about the longest road trip you have ever taken. (It is alright if you have never taken any long trips. Just pull up Google Maps and see how far it is, both in miles and hours, from the east coast to the west coast on I-10.) This is not about how you traveled, but about getting your mind in the right place so you are ready for ***THIS*** journey.

Ok, so the farthest I have ever traveled is to Zimbabwe on the African continent. The first leg of the flight is sixteen hours. The second leg is ten hours, and the final leg is three hours. Sounds pretty brutal, doesn't it? Sixteen hours on a plane? The total travel time is about 34 hours. YIKES!

When we start talking about taking a trip, we usually talk about what day and time we are going to leave. Since we are traveling by car, we must decide if we are going to rent a car or drive our own. We also must decide when are we going to put gas in the car and who is going to drive first.

Lots of thought and planning go into taking a trip. We need to get an idea about where we will stop for gas and snacks. (If you are driving in Texas, you look to see where the next Buc-ee's is.) We don't often talk about the people or the activities. The destination tends to be our focus. While we are planning, we are strictly thinking about leaving from point A and arriving at point B. No other descriptions of our trip exist.

But, honestly, is the trip about the city we are going to? *WHY* did we really get in that car in the first place? (There is that whole *why* thing again.) *WHY* did we decide we really needed to make this trip? Are we running a race that is over as soon as we cross the city limits? Can we go back home as soon as we arrive?

What I realized is when I am going somewhere, it is not about the somewhere or the name of the destination. I realized the reason I could sit on that airplane for sixteen hours of flight time (that does not include the before takeoff and after landing time) had nothing to do with the airport on the other end. The reason I could sit in the car for about eighteen hours had nothing to do with the city on the other end. It had everything to do with whom I was going to spend time, what we were going to do, and the memories we were going to create. Those things are *why* I got on the plane and in the car and traveled the distance. Those things (my ***WHY***) made it possible for me to sit that long.

Now, let's look at this journey in a bit more detail and see how it will relate to *your* weight loss journey.

Focus is not on the end

Unless we own a plane and fly it ourselves, a lot of the trip is out of our control. Even a lot is out of our control when we drive our own car. Ok, the only things that are actually in our control are when we leave the house and what we pack in our suitcase—and other things can affect even that. The rest we must adapt to as we make quick decisions and exercise patience.

So, you have taken the time to decide *why* taking this trip is important. You have decided to take a journey to love yourself and change your relationship with food, which will undoubtedly result in weight loss. And you are about to leave your house.

Wait! Consider what else you did before you took your longest trip ever. Didn't you make some plans and pack your bag? Didn't you ask the neighbors to water your plants and take care of your pet goldfish? Didn't you contact the post office and ask them to hold your mail? Didn't you make sure you had the right clothes, the right shoes, and all the other right stuff you needed once you arrived? (Yes, I know most places have a Walmart, but trust me, I have traveled to places, even in the US, where Walmart was not that close by.)

So, you must plan, prepare, and pack your bag for this journey before you leave the house.

Look through your pantry and fridge and toss out or give away anything that might cause a traffic jam or delay or go bad while you are gone. For me to be successful, I had to keep those things out of the house. Now, I know other people probably live with you in your house. Other people lived in my house too. Trust me, even if you have kids, you can replace candy, cookies, and crackers with fruit and cheese. They will adapt. (Remember the oxygen mask you packed? Here is one place you can use it.)
Ok, you have packed your bags and emptied the trash. We are almost ready to go.

> A traffic jam is any food, occasion, celebration, or even person that can stop your journey to filling that *myself*-sized hole in your heart.

Get out your map (your ***WHY***). I like to look at maps because I like to know where I am going and what interesting things I might see along the way. I like to know how far apart the towns are on my trip. (I live in Texas. We measure distance in hours, not miles. For example, it can take an hour to get across Houston. 😉)

Now, this journey is NOT about the destination; it is about *the journey*. But you still need to have an idea of where you are headed. If you don't know your destination, how will you know when you have arrived? On the back of your ***WHY*** statement, write down your ***weight destination*** in *very small print*. If you want to know about how many calories your body needs each day go to info.youcanteatlove.com (You can also write it in your workbook – the very last page, the very last line.) Remember, this journey is not about the destination. On this journey, our focus will be on the next mile marker on the highway, the next stop, and the beautiful sights we see along the way. Eventually, we will reach our destination.

OK, it's time to leave. Load your bags into the car. Double-check to make sure you turned off all the lights. Tell your pet goldfish you will see him soon and hop in the car.

Off we go!

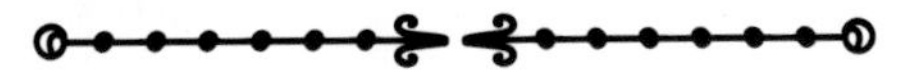

What's in your suitcase?

- Trash bags
- Oxygen mask
- ***WHY***
- Friedrich Nietzsche quote
- Photo of you
- Index cards
- Stake
- Hammer
- website

- Snap a photo – post it to the You Can't Eat Love Facebook page
- Join the private You Can't Eat Love Facebook group
- Workbook
- *So, I said to myself...* Journal
- Pens
- Highlighters

Life Hacks

- The greatest gift you can give yourself as you begin this journey is to clean out your pantry, fridge, and freezer. Get rid of any foods that cause problems for you. Make a list of some fresh items you can substitute for what you're eliminating and make a quick trip to the store. Only pick up what is on your list.

Jackie Says

- Don't skip warmups
- Remember, results take time

Weblinks

https://linktr.ee/youcanteatlove

SECTION II

I AM SEEKING TO FIND YOU

Never, never, never give up.
Winston Churchill

CHAPTER 5

If It Were Easy, Everyone Would Do It

Healing doesn't mean the damage never existed.
It means the damage no longer controls our lives.
Shah Rukh Khan

People, people needing people?

When you told someone about a trip you had planned, have they ever said, "Why are you going there? You should be going here. Or, you shouldn't be going at all." (I promised we would talk about that "sh" word, and we will, just not yet.) Frustrating, isn't it? Especially when you try to explain WHY you plan on going there. After your very well-thought-out explanation, they still don't understand and still think you should go somewhere else. Or they think you shouldn't go anywhere at all. You should just stay right there.

Well, guess what? On this trip, we (you and I together equal we) are not going to discuss any of the details of our trip with anyone. In fact, we are not even going to *tell* anyone we are taking a trip. We are going to pack our bags, go and just wonder how long it will take before someone notices things are changing.

Now, I can already hear the thoughts spinning in your head. *Why would I not tell people I am going on a diet?* Well, how many times have you told someone about your intention to lose weight? How did the conversation go over lunch or while you were enjoying a snack after dinner? How about when you went to the movies? How did you *honestly* feel about the comments made regarding your choice?

Right now, I want you to get out your pen and workbook and write down the things that were said to you when you told someone you were going on a diet. Write down how you felt when you heard their response. Then, I want you to write down what you did next and *how you felt*. Be honest. I will wait.

Were you surprised at what you discovered?

This trip is a *little different*, which is *why* we are *not* telling anyone about it. You are **not** going on a diet. From this moment forward, you do not have to use that awful four-letter word again. You are changing your relationship with food. You are discovering and learning how to live a different lifestyle—a lifestyle that lines up with *your* ***WHY***. This new lifestyle is *how* you are going to bring your ***WHY*** to life.

I hated (yes, hated) having someone question my choice of food or snack. I felt like the diet police were sitting at the table with me, questioning whether I should be having that hamburger, stuffed potato, or piece of pie. I could feel two emotions rising inside of me. One was anger. How dare this person question my food choice? The second emotion was shame. Maybe I should not be eating this. Then all of that would set off another set of problems. I would eat whatever that food was "just to show them." Honestly though, who was I showing?

You—and doing something about you

On our journey together, we are going to learn a lot about ourselves and how changing our thoughts changes our relationship with food. I want to provide you with a shortcut to something that took me a long time to learn: *I can only do something about me*. You can only do something about you.

Remember that oxygen mask you packed? Here is where it comes into play. Your ***WHY*** for this journey is **about you** and not about the other people in your life. They are on their own. Will they benefit from your journey? Yes, they will because you *will* enjoy a healthier, happier life.

But for this journey, you come first. What is in your best interest comes first. So, put on your oxygen mask first. Put on your oxygen mask when you are around people who are not helping you on your journey.

This journey is a *me* thing, not a *we* thing (unless of course, it is about you and me). This is a journey each of us travels alone, even though we are doing it together. None of us are on the same path. None of us are arriving at the same destination. Alone together, not together alone.

I will show you how to become your best friend, so you are never alone without someone positive in your life. You will learn to speak your kindest words to yourself. When you need to hear encouraging words from someone, just stop by (you can email me at leslie@youcanteatlove.com or post a message in the closed Facebook group You Can't Eat Love). I will tell you how amazing you are and how proud I am of you.

You can come into this circle and share because *we* know the rules. The rules are cheers, hugs, kind words, nods, shared tears, and smiles. Nothing else. No negative comments or "shoulds" are allowed.

Anyone need a battery charger?

Have you ever noticed that negative and "shoulding" people drain your energy? The more you allow them to drain you by giving them permission to comment on your decision or choice, the less you will be able to hold on to your ***WHY***. You need your ***WHY*** to help keep you on the journey when you want to give up. Do not let other people be the reason you give up.

You worked hard on your ***WHY***. Protect it and keep it shining in front of you. Look at it every day.

Stop and look at your ***WHY*** right now. It is not a sleeping baby; it is a full-of-energy teenager. Your ***WHY*** is loaded with action and possibilities.

Another hard thing you will run into on this journey (and another reason to not discuss it with anyone) is sabotaging people. You know who I am talking about. In my house, it's my husband.

No matter how many times I ask my husband to not give me anything chocolate for my birthday, he will bring home not one, not two, but three different chocolate cheesecake things. He will buy large bags of Kisses or Snickers or ice cream. He refuses to accept those things talk to me and are not safe anywhere near me.

I keep telling my husband the chocolates, ice cream, etc. do not know how to behave. They call my name and jump out of their containers and into my mouth before I can get away. He will comment something like "Just have one bite and move on." But for me, it does not work quite that way.

Do you have a "well-meaning" parent or friend who insists that a little won't hurt you? How many times has this "well-meaning" person told you they made it just for you or Aunt So and So would be so hurt if you did not...(I put well-meaning in quotes, because truthfully if they had your best interest in mind, they would listen to your first gentle refusal and move on instead of insisting.)

What these people refuse to accept is that a little bit will hurt you. (We will talk about that more shortly.) And I can tell you from personal experience, they will not change no matter how well you explain yourself.

Saboteurs are like wolves in sheep's clothing. They masquerade as kind and innocent. But be aware of them. People who insist on us eating things we do not want are food pushers—not "kind souls."

Take a moment to make a list of the saboteurs and "kind souls" in your life. You can write this in your workbook. You will soon see these people do not have your best interest at heart.

We will practice dealing with these people in just a bit. You can work on forming responses and action plans for each one. You need to be prepared for your next encounter. You don't want them to pull you out of your car. Road rash is not pretty.

Here we go to the next tough thing. *You* can be one of your own saboteurs. How many times have you told yourself just one bag of chips or one slice of cake won't hurt you? How many times have you told yourself you will walk a few more minutes so you can eat those cookies? How about the promises you make that tomorrow you will "get back on your diet"? (I will tell you another secret – tomorrow never arrives; there is only the present and the past) What you say to yourself is *just as important* as what other people say to you.

Start noticing when you are saying unkind things to yourself. If you want, you can list these unkind things or make notes to yourself on paper or in the filing cabinet in your mind. The key is to notice the unkind things you say to yourself and switch them to kind things.

What you fill your mind with is what you fill your heart with—and that is what eventually comes out of your mouth. So, speaking kindly to yourself will start to fill your heart and the *myself*-sized hole will begin getting just a tiny bit smaller.

I have a book of positive thoughts I read every morning. This jump-starts the positive conversations I have with myself. Find one you like and toss it into your suitcase.

I would love to hear from you how you feel about speaking kindly to yourself. What are you telling yourself?

- On this journey, you will get comfortable putting you and your needs first.
- Do something about you.
- Have a plan for dealing with sabotaging people and "kind souls" in your life.
- What you are saying to yourself is just as important as what other people are saying to you. Start saying to yourself things like the following:
    - "I am a person who eats fruit."
    - "I am a person who eats boneless, skinless breast of chicken."
    - "I am a person who can politely accept and dispose of food I have chosen to not eat."
    - "I am a person who plans and follows my plan to the best of my ability."
- There is no room in your life for shame. You are filling the "*myself*"-sized hole in your heart with love.

We keep going back to the only person you can do anything about—and that is you. Be true to yourself. You have your ***WHY***; keep it close. Oxygen mask on.

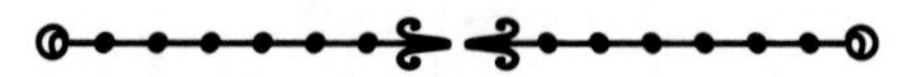

What's in your suitcase?

- Idea about your destination
- Plan for saboteurs
- Plan for food pushers
- Trash bags
- Oxygen mask
- ***WHY***
- Friedrich Nietzsche quote
- Photo of you
- Index cards
- Stake
- Hammer
- website
- Snap a photo – post it to the You Can't Eat Love Facebook page
- Join the private You Can't Eat Love Facebook group
- Workbook
- *So, I said to myself...*Journal
- Pens
- Highlighters

Life Hacks

- Alone together, not together alone. Remember.

Jackie Says

- Do workouts you enjoy
- Think of exercise as taking great care of yourself and not punishment

Weblinks

https://linktr.ee/youcanteatlove

CHAPTER 6

I'm Going to Cry If I Want to

When everything seems to be against you, remember that the airplane takes off against the wind, not with it.

Henry Ford

Planes, trains—we are traveling by automobile

So, here we are, off on our grand adventure. Now, just like on any other trip you have ever taken, we are going to run into some problems. Just like with any other trip, we need to think about what the problems might be and how we can keep them from stopping us on our journey.

I live in a smallish town outside of the city limits of Houston. Around here, one city/town blends into the other. Not too many clear boundary lines exist.

> *What we do have are lots of freeways. The world's widest section of freeway runs from downtown Houston to my town. As a matter of fact, this section of I-10 is named after my town, Katy. I-10 is so wide it can be seen from space.*

I want you to think about your journey like the closest freeway/highway. I want you to visualize that stretch of road. If you need to see it closer, pull it up on Google Maps. What I want you to see is that freeway or highway is not straight. (Yes, I realize some stretches of highways are very long and straight but humor me and look a little further down the road.) In a lot of places, that freeway is not even flat.

The freeway is a picture of what your journey will look like. The journey is not going to be straight, and it definitely ***will not*** be flat. In some places, the road goes up, and in other places, it goes down. The important thing is the road takes you where you are going. Remember, this is about the journey, not the destination.

I try to stay off the freeway during rush hour. The traffic jams can be a bit frustrating. Sometimes, you can sit still and not move at all for a while. Sometimes, you just inch forward a little at a time.

Have you ever been stuck in a traffic jam and just parked your car, gotten out, and walked home? Neither have I. Why? Because I know eventually the traffic will clear, and I will be able to get to where I am going.

There will be times during your journey when you will consider giving up because you don't see the kind of progress you would like to. *That* is when I want you to think about the last time you were stuck in a traffic jam. What did you *do*?

I bet you did not park your car, get out, and walk home. I don't do that either when I am stuck in a traffic jam. What I do is find a song on the radio or my phone and sing loudly. Or I call someone I have not had the time to call and chat with. What I **<u>don't</u>** do, is park my car, get out and walk home.

Let's start planning now for the traffic jams we are going to run into on this journey. Grab your pen and workbook again. (You thought I was going to do all the writing?)
Let's think about some things we can do so we are not tempted to park the car and walk home. To get your creative juices flowing, I will share a couple of easy things with you. Add a five- to ten-minute walk to your day. Change your mid-afternoon snack from a banana to an apple.

Now it's your turn. What will you do to avoid parking your car? Go on. I will wait.

Your traveling companion

Before we get too far down the road, I want you to meet the most important person you have with you on this journey. You. Yes, you. (If you double-check your suitcase, you will find yourself in there.)

Let's think about this. Who is the one person that is always right there? Who is the one person carrying on conversations with you even when they should be quiet?

You.

Like on any journey, you will get to know your traveling companions. You will get to know *you* very well. You will become your very best friend.

A mind is a terrible maze to waste

Think back to the last time you made a promise to yourself to not eat something. What was it?

Chips were the most recent thing I promised to not eat. Chips (like almost anything chocolate) are my kryptonite. On occasion, I will catch myself having eaten a bag or two. Since it is just us, I will be very honest with you. Sometimes it's three or four. (We have that many available at once because my husband likes the multi-packs of chips so he can have a bag or two with his lunch or just for a snack.)

When I come to consciousness, I start having a conversation with myself that goes something like this:

> *"What were you thinking? You know you only planned to have one bag of chips! What is going on? Why can't you just make your plan and stick to it?"*

And then the shame starts.

Have you ever done that? In your workbook, write down those conversations you have with yourself. Read, out loud, what you wrote down. I want you to hear the words you are saying and feel what you are feeling. Write down what you are feeling.

Now, I want you to read that same conversation again, ***but this time***, I want you to shout "**STOP**!" (You can say it out loud if you want to. I do if I am by myself) Shout it again.

Now, imagine you are hearing your very best friend in the whole world having a shame-filled conversation with themselves. You would not want your BFF to feel the shame you felt earlier, would you? What would you say to them?

> *"It's ok you ate the chips. I know you had a plan. Sometimes plans work and sometimes they don't. I am curious why the plan didn't work this time. ("I am curious" is a very neutral phrase. Try using it with yourself and a couple of people around you. Observe the response. If you want, you can share on the You Can't Eat Love Facebook page.) Is there something going on you want to talk about? What do you think you might do differently next time?"*

Notice what you say to your BFF is probably a lot kinder than what you say to yourself. But our goal is not perfection. You can practice being kind to yourself too.

Here is a big secret: *listen* to what you have to say next in response to the questions you asked your BFF. If it's easier, write down the conversation you would have with your BFF. (I carry on all kinds of written conversations with myself all the time. This makes it easier for me to focus.) Be honest; that's how we grow.

Eating unplanned food is just a traffic jam on the journey. Remember to change the radio station or phone a friend. You can even work your way off the freeway so you can move forward on the surface streets. But do not park your car, get out, and walk home.

Go ahead and add "STOP" to your suitcase. This is almost as important as your oxygen mask.

Batteries in the remote control need to be replaced

Changing our beliefs and thoughts is the most powerful part of changing our relationship with food. Accepting our imperfections and forgiveness are key aspects of our new way of thinking. I am not just talking about forgiving others but also forgiving yourself.

How easy is it for you to forgive someone when they have done something that hurts you? How easy is it to forgive yourself? You *can learn* to acknowledge when you do mess up, calm yourself, and then get up and keep going.

Practice forgiving yourself. Release yourself from thinking you must be perfect or anything else. You just have to *be*. That's all, nothing else.

Remember the bag of chips we were talking about earlier? As soon as you come to consciousness that you were eating unplanned food *and* you listen to *why* you were eating it, I want you to tell yourself "I forgive you."

You don't need to say what for or why, simply say "I forgive you" and mean it.

Sit in that forgiveness for a moment. Feel the release of shame and the increase of self-love. Enjoy the feeling. This is one of the memories that will help you on your journey. You will bring it to mind time and again. Think traffic jam. Don't park the car. Don't get out. Don't walk home.

You are probably curious why I said "come to consciousness" you were eating unplanned food. I have come to believe I must give myself the benefit of the doubt. I know I had a plan and all intentions of executing the plan. So, the only explanation for my not-so-great choice is I slipped into a lack of consciousness while awake. In other words, I slid back into a bad habit.

Sliding back into bad habits does not feel good. So, instead, I choose to give myself some grace and say, "I slipped into an awake lack of consciousness." No shame. No should. Only encouraging, helpful, and kind thoughts. Do not give yourself an excuse to park the car, get out, and walk home.

Let's take a moment to talk more about habits. We create habits when we do stuff over and over again. They can be good habits, helpful habits, or destructive habits. Good and bad habits are all created the same way.

Think of a habit as a car that is driven down a muddy road every day. The muddy road develops ruts, and each time the car goes down the road, the ruts get a little deeper. Pretty soon, you have a self-driving car because the ruts are so deep, the car must stay in them. Do you see how a habit can become a self-driving car?

To create a new habit, you must keep driving your car down the muddy road, the exact same muddy road as your other habits. Maybe your new habit will be making your favorite sandwich with one slice of bread instead of two. Just because you are driving in a new spot, does not mean the ruts have gone away. The ruts are filling up slowly—very slowly—but they are still there. If you inch too far to one side or the other, your new car is going to fall into the old ruts, and you will have to climb out.

Does this mean you are doomed to struggle driving your new car down the muddy road? No. Each time you successfully complete a trip, your new ruts get a little deeper and the old ones fill up a little more.

Each time you successfully drive your car down that muddy road, I want you to give yourself a big cheer. Throw in a few stickers while you are at it! If you feel like you cannot get out of the old ruts, just let me know and we will figure it out together. Remember, you are part of a community.

I also see habits I am trying to eliminate as scary monsters I have trapped in the basement. I have about ten different locks to make certain the door is secure and none of the monsters can get out.

Sometimes, I go down into the basement to get one of those monsters so I can try to tame it (crazy, I know), and I forget to lock all ten of the locks. Forgetting to lock even one lock makes it easy for the monsters to get out and take over again. Like the genie that escapes from the bottle, the monsters are harder to put back in than they were to put in the basement the first time.

If you have trouble putting all those monsters back in the basement (or cellar), just holler. I will help you put all those monsters back in so they cannot get out. I will even brace the door while you lock ALL the locks. You are worth it.

> I don't want you to make a list of all the times you're not kind to yourself, *I do* want you to start noticing when you're catching unkind thoughts and switching them to kind thoughts. You can make notes to yourself on paper, or in the filing cabinet you have in your mind. Either way, notice. Soon, you'll notice how many times a day you're saying kind things to yourself. An enormously powerful lesson is this – what you're filling your mind with is what you're filling your heart with and that's what comes out of your mouth. So, speaking kindly to yourself will start to fill your heart and the *"myself"* sized hole will begin getting just a tiny bit smaller. I would love to hear from you how you feel about speaking kindly to yourself. I would love to hear what you're telling yourself. I have a book of positive thoughts I read every morning. This jump starts the positive conversations I have with myself. Find one you like and toss it into your suitcase.

Not all families are created equal

I am going to tell you another secret. Your family helped form your initial relationship with food. Where I lived growing up, the number of people in my family, my mom's dislike for food, and our situation influenced my first relationship with food. We lived out of the country in camps for American employees and their families. The only place to shop for groceries was a commissary. It had limited options because most of the non-perishable foods had to be imported. After we moved back to the States, we lived in a small town and the closest major grocery was over 20 miles away. Not too easy for a quick run to the store. We were not poor; it was just difficult to either get a variety of groceries or be able to store large amounts, so my mom prioritized what she bought at the store and strictly portioned everything.

Because I grew up where someone else portioned the food and made the decisions about how much I could eat, I didn't learn to portion my own food or stop eating after I was satisfied. When I was in a buffet or a serve yourself situation, I didn't know what a normal-sized portion should look like. I didn't know I could savor food and stop eating before I felt like I was going to burst. (Savor and savory were unfamiliar words to me. I was only familiar with salt and pepper for seasoning food.)

I did not develop self-control.

I didn't learn how to enjoy "special" foods because so many foods were "special." If a food we rarely had was available, I had zero self-control. I believed I would never get it again.

I did learn how to divide by eight.

I remember visiting one of my friends who would have chips and onion dip at their house. I thought I had struck gold. I didn't understand what one of her brothers was actually telling me when he would call me the "onion dip queen." I just thought he was making a joking comment. What he was telling me was he noticed how much onion dip I was eating. Shame washed over me when I recalled all those times I ate chips and onion dip at their house.

I still recall the first time I went through the dorm cafeteria line at college. You can go back for seconds? Really? Oh my. Forget the freshman fifteen. I passed that mark long before the first week of classes was over. Do you have any memories like that?

I had to have a lot of conversations with myself to unlearn these behaviors. I had to tell myself I could go to the store and get more, just not right now. I learned to be kind to myself and understand where my feelings about food were coming from. I had to drive my new car to make new ruts. It took a lot of work, a lot of forgiving myself, and a lot of patience with myself. But just like you, I am worth it. I was filling the *myself*-sized hole in my heart, little by little.

Take a moment, in your workbook, to write down your family's philosophy about food. I want you to really think about the relationship your family had with snacks, special occasions, and just everyday meals. You might be surprised at what you discover. I was.

This is a process of discovery and understanding where our food relationship comes from. We cannot change our relationship with food unless we understand it. One of my favorite quotes is from the cartoon *GI Joe*: "Now you know and knowing is half the battle." Uncovering this information will help you stay in the car and not walk home. Understanding your family's philosophy about food will also help you prepare for and participate in your next family gathering.

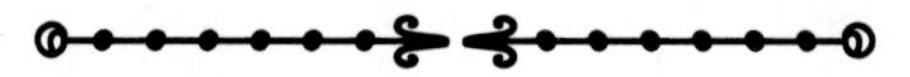

What's in your suitcase?

- Google maps
- Locks
- "Traffic Jam" written on an index card
- From www.youcanteatlove.com print off the "Stay" card
- Book of positive affirmations
- Seasoning
- Forgiveness
- Choices

- Community
- Stop
- Idea about your destination
- Plan for saboteurs
- Plan for food pushers
- Trash bags
- Oxygen mask
- ***WHY***
- Friedrich Nietzsche quote
- Photo of you
- Index cards
- Stake
- Hammer
- website
- Snap a photo – post it to the You Can't Eat Love Facebook page
- Join the private You Can't Eat Love Facebook group
- Workbook
- *So, I said to myself...*Journal
- Pens
- Highlighters

Life Hacks

- You just have to be
- Choose – don't give away your power

Jackie says

- Fall in love with the process
- Don't weigh every day

Weblinks

https://linktr.ee/youcanteatlove

CHAPTER 7

No Should Zone

Do something today that your future self will thank you for tomorrow.

Sean Patrick Flanery

Let's talk about word choices. My least favorite saying is "Sticks and stones may break my bones, but words will never hurt me." This is a very untrue statement. Words will and do hurt. They can do indescribable damage as they run around in our heads, replaying the same tune like a song stuck on repeat.

A simple word has more power than a traffic jam. A simple word can cause you to park your car, get out, and ***run*** home. So, we need to eliminate some words to help us keep going on our journey.

Remember, earlier, I said we would talk about "should"? Well, here we are. Let's talk about this awful word and take its power away. (You will find a section in your workbook on should, shouldn't, and shoulding.)

How many times have you had a conversation with yourself that started something like this: "I should have..." (You fill in the blank.) How many times did your sentences sound like mine? "I should have had only one piece of cake instead of two." "I should have had the carrots instead of the chips."

How do you feel when you either hear or say those "should's" and "shouldn'ts?" Is there a difference in how you feel when someone else says these words to you versus when you say them to yourself? We have a hard enough time not "shoulding" ourselves. Do we need to give that power to someone else?

Truthfully, changing your relationship with food is less about the food and more about what is going on in your head. You know, those internal conversations. To be honest, there are no "bad" foods or foods you "shouldn't" eat unless you have a health condition that requires a restricted diet.

Should is one of those subtle shaming words. Webster's Dictionary defines "should" as "used to indicate obligation, duty, or correctness, typically when criticizing someone's actions". (Webster, 1988) Criticizing *your* actions. Criticizing *your* choice in what you eat.

Pay attention to how often you use "should" when talking to yourself. Listen to how often you hear others using it. Notice how you feel. In your workbook, list the times you "should" all over yourself and list the people who "should" on you. (Once I started noticing how often "should" was used, it became like a red car, or whatever color or make your first car was. I heard it everywhere.)

We will practice getting into the "No should" zone. Start listening for the word. When someone else uses it when they are speaking to you, reframe their sentence and repeat it back without the "sh" word in it.

> "Dear, you really should not eat that piece of cake." Reframe it and repeat back to them "I am making a choice to eat this piece of cake." You see, keep your power. Let them know (politely) they have trespassed into your territory. Another of my favorites (and why I did not tell anyone I had gone on this journey) is "Should you eat those french fries? I thought you were on a diet." "It is my choice to eat these french fries." Think about these examples and come up with a few of your own. You can explore this a bit more in the workbook.

What's in your suitcase?

- No Should Zone t-shirt and poster
- Your power
- Google maps
- Locks
- "Traffic Jam" written on an index card
- Print off the "Stay" card
- Book of positive affirmations
- Seasoning
- Forgiveness
- Choices
- Community
- Stop
- Idea about your destination
- Plan for saboteurs
- Plan for food pushers
- Trash bags
- Oxygen mask
- ***WHY***
- Friedrich Nietzsche quote
- Photo of you
- Index cards
- Stake
- Hammer
- website
- Snap a photo – post it to the You Can't Eat Love Facebook page
- Join the private You Can't Eat Love Facebook group
- Workbook
- *So, I said to myself...*Journal
- Pens
- Highlighters

Life Hacks

- Reframing comments we make to ourselves helps keep our car driving forward in those new ruts on that muddy road
- How many times did you hear a phrase that went something like this "you should (see that ugly word?) be ashamed of yourself." Think about how

you felt. Delete that phrase – you are wonderful, kind, smart, and beautiful. Nowhere in the description of you is shame.

- Toss "shame" out of the window along with "ashamed". Positive words filling your mind will help you on this journey.

Jackie says

- Drink lots of water!

Weblinks

https://linktr.ee/youcanteatlove

CHAPTER 8

Back To Our Regularly Scheduled Program

I can only do me. Everyone else has to do them.

Leslie Lindsey Davis

You are probably getting a bit tired of me mentioning feelings. (That would be a great song. Oh, wait. It is. Morris Alpert wrote and sang it.). You are probably wondering when I am going to get to the losing weight part of this book.

Well, here is a little secret I learned. Losing weight is a diet—a short-term fix. What you and I are doing is discovering ***WHY*** we need to lose weight so we can return to our real self. We are healing the broken parts, so we don't need a temporary fix like food; which was my "drug of choice." Little by little, the healing fills the *myself*-sized hole in our heart.

You will never be the same as you were when you started this journey—and that is something worth cheering for. I want you to take just a moment to stand up and cheer as loudly as you can. Cheer for you! See how great that feels? (And there are those feelings again. Yes, a lot of our relationship with food is connected to feelings.) If you like, share with the group on Facebook so we can cheer for you too!

The hard work of returning to our real self is about looking at our thoughts and feelings. This is not easy. (It is so much easier to use food to fill the *myself*-sized hole in our heart.)

This part of our journey will make us the best we can be when we arrive at our stopping point. Here is some exciting news.

The stopping point is also the starting point for a new journey to the rest of your amazing life.

So, hang in here with me. Feelings are tough. Thoughts are tough. Relationships are tough. But together, we will figure this out. Promise me you will not park your car. You will not get out. And you will not walk home.

Lies and more lies

True confession time. Before I began this journey, I hated feelings. I believed feelings were signs of weakness. Feelings were very messy.

Growing up, I had no idea there was a long list of things I *could* feel. I knew the names of these feelings and could describe them. I just did not know I was allowed to *feel* them.

I did master two feelings: anger and sadness. But I cannot say that I was ever genuinely happy. I know, I know. It sounds so dramatic, but it is true. I was not unhappy, just not content, happy, and smiling all the time.

Truthfully, it is ok I was not happy. I recognize my parents did the best they could. Now I am an adult, I can choose to do things differently—so I do.

I learned my feelings will not kill me. It is ok to feel sad or mad or even joyful. By getting acquainted with my feelings, I have loosened the ties food had on them.

Before being brave enough to feel sad, I would search everywhere—the pantry, the refrigerator, and the freezer—looking for "something." I did not understand food was my "drug of choice." Eating was how I killed the pain of honest feelings because *I was afraid of feeling*.

The insanity of trying to stop my feelings with food was the flood of guilt, shame, and negative self-talk that followed. Remember the four-year-old throwing a temper tantrum? That four-year-old has a parent. That parent—the harsh, critical, judging, shaming parent—would show up when I used my "drug of choice."

How about you? How do you cope with your genuine emotions? In your workbook, start listing your emotions and how you deal with them. Be honest about who shows up in your mind. If it gets too scary, reach out either in the Facebook group or by email (leslie@youcanteatlove.com). Remember, we are on this journey together; it's not just you, alone.

Little by little, I allowed myself to sit in whatever emotion I was feeling. Sometimes, it was for five minutes. Sometimes, it was for only five seconds. This did not happen overnight, but it did happen.

I learned to not run from my feelings. Deciding to not get out of the car was so important when I sat in my emotions. I knew I could change the radio. I could go outside for just a moment. I could call or text someone. I could do something different, *and* I would be ok.

Then, when the moment passed, I would tell myself how proud I was of myself. I was filling that *myself*-sized hole in my heart with love for myself. I was not allowing anyone or anything to make the hole deeper.

Go back to the list of your emotions in your workbook. Think about what you can do the next time a scary feeling or emotion starts washing over you. I want you to be prepared. Think about what you are going to tell yourself when you succeed in staying in the car. The workbook has some examples to help you get started. (This is when your BFFITWWW shows up. 😊)

See, you are moving forward, mile by mile.

My least favorite commercials are the ones where someone is sad, and another person offers them some treat to help them feel better. Think about the message that sends. Wouldn't it be better to just sit with the person, ask them if they want to talk, and then just listen? (I'm probably not very popular with the snack food people. 😉)

Food does not make emotional pain or those scary emotions go away. Food is not the same as a warm bear-hug and a sincere "I love you, and I can only imagine how you must feel." I hope you are seeing that food will not fill the *myself*-sized hole in your heart, no matter how many forkfuls you try to cram in.

Let's break that chain of using food to solve our emotional problems by learning to love ourselves so we can sincerely love the people around us. Let's break the chain by not being afraid to feel and naming our feelings. And then, let's be kind to ourselves.

Who are you really lying to?

Have you ever lied to yourself about what you are going to eat and how much you ate? I tell myself I am going to have five crackers, and before I have turned around twice, I have eaten ten or more crackers, but I keep telling myself I only had five. Now, crackers are not going to make or break my journey—but the lie I tell myself will. (Believe me when I tell you I went through a lot of lightbulbs on this journey. I probably should have bought stock in the lightbulb manufacturer.)

One day, it occurred to me there were only two people in the whole wide world I could lie to. I could only lie to me and myself. "I" sees everything.

> *I can hear you saying, "Now, wait a minute. What do you mean you can only lie to me and myself? What about the other people in your life? You can lie to them." My answer is: "not really." The other people in my life and the other people in your life see the evidence of our choices. As they (this time we know who these they people are) say in all the lawyer shows, the evidence speaks for itself.*

So, back to the lying to me and myself. The mind is a very powerful, living thing. If we tell our mind enough lies, it will take them as truth.

The sooner we get honest with me and myself, the easier it is to stay in the car. Me and myself do not like hard work. They want things to be easy. Me and myself are the ones hollering for the "miracle pill."

As much as I did not like it, I had to get honest and tell me and myself it was going to be ok. We will talk later about some of the tricks I used.

For right now, in your workbook, I want you to make a list of the lies you are telling yourself. I will share some of mine with you. Here they are:

- These pants are only supposed to go to my ankles.
- That chair is made from flimsy material.
- My eyes look squinty because I am looking into the sun.

- → I don't have a double chin; my head was tilted wrong.
- → I have no idea what happened to all the cookies.

Once you make a list of the lies you are telling yourself, forgive me and myself for trying to protect you. Tell them you will be ok; you are ready to see yourself just as you are. Me and myself truly do care about you. They just want your life to be as painless as possible.

You've got this. You really are ready to stay in the car and not walk home. Remember, *you are never alone.*

Now, to show me and myself how brave you are, go stand in front of a full-length mirror and take a picture of yourself. You don't have to look at the photo now. Look at it when you are ready.

But do save the photo in a special album on your phone. You could call that album "My Journey Back to Me." You will be taking lots of pictures of yourself. I don't want you to make the mistake I did. Finding my photos was an ordeal since I had them scattered all over my phone. (I do need a smack my head emoji here. 😉) The important thing is keeping a record of the beginning of your journey, just like you would for any other trip.

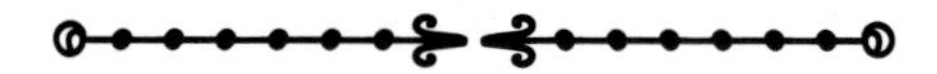

What's in your suitcase?

- Megaphone (for louder cheering!)
- Tissues
- Full-length photo
- Album set up in your phone or on your computer where you will store your "becoming you" photos

- No Should Zone t-shirt and poster
- Your power
- Google maps
- Locks
- "Traffic Jam" written on an index card
- Print off the "Stay" card
- Book of positive affirmations
- Seasoning
- Forgiveness
- Choices
- Community
- Stop
- Idea about your destination
- Plan for saboteurs
- Plan for food pushers
- Trash bags
- Oxygen mask
- ***WHY***
- Friedrich Nietzsche quote
- Photo of you
- Index cards
- Stake
- Hammer
- website
- Snap a photo – post it to the You Can't Eat Love Facebook page
- Join the private You Can't Eat Love Facebook group
- Workbook
- *So, I said to myself...*Journal
- Pens
- Highlighter

Life Hacks

- "Oh, well" became a phrase I used when I would make not-so-great choices that I did not want to make. Sometimes the emotions would override my logic and as soon as I understood what had happened, I would say "oh, well" instead of beating myself up. Sometimes, "oh, well" is all I could get out. I prefer to forgive myself but sometimes, "oh, well" is enough.

Jackie says

- Be consistent
- Make a date with yourself

Weblinks

https://linktr.ee/youcanteatlove

CHAPTER 9

Cheater, Cheater, Pumpkin Eater

Love yourself first, and everything else falls in line.
You really have to love yourself to get anything done in this world.

Lucille Ball

Before I understood I needed to change my relationship with food and no diet in the world was the answer to my losing weight, I would say to myself (and sometimes to other people), "I cheated on my diet." Really? Who did I "cheat" on? I cannot tell you the exact moment the board smacked me between the eyes, but I do recall a lot of lightbulbs turning on. (See, I told you I should have bought stock. Where is the smack my head emoji when you need it?)

Think about the word cheat. Truthfully, there are only three ways we can cheat—on a test, on a relationship, or our taxes. Anything else is simply an alternate reality. Something we are pretending is something else.

How many times have you heard someone talk about a "cheat" day? How about a "cheat" snack? This is another lie I told myself. Having a cheat day, cheat snack, cheat meal, or any cheat food is not a "cheat" at all. ***It is just a choice.***

Please, remove the word cheat from your vocabulary when you are talking about food. That one word takes your power away. You do have power over food. Toss "cheat" out of the window of your car and keep moving forward. We don't care if "cheat" gets road rash.

A lot of what we are talking about comes back around to words, which have the power to help us or to harm us.

The more positive self-talk we have, the less room there is for negative garbage. It's better to lose some words that will not help us on this journey or the next one. (Think of how many new words you are picking up. Check your suitcase and make sure it will still zip!)

Our minds are very powerful, and we believe the words we feed our minds. On this journey, we are forming some new beliefs. We are learning to be kind to ourselves and to forgive ourselves. We are driving new cars down new ruts, so we also form new habits. We are becoming our very own best cheerleader.

We are going to reclaim our power. And I am not talking about willpower. Will power carries the heavy weight of shaming and should. In any talk about willpower, there is no room for kindness, grace, or forgiveness, which we need a lot of on this journey. So, if you have been dragging willpower around with you, toss it out the window of your car; right behind cheat.

I want you to think about everything as a choice. When we have choices and can make choices, we have power. Isn't a lot of your relationship with food about not having power? Isn't part of the *myself*-sized hole in your heart because you gave away your power, hoping to get something back?

There are three kinds of choices for food. The first is a great choice such as deciding to have your salad dressing on the side. The second is a good choice like deciding to eat two cookies instead of four. The third is a not-so-great choice such as deciding you are going to eat the pasta on your kids' plates. There are no other types of choices.

In your workbook, make notes of when you have told yourself you were cheating with food. Then for each instance, I want you to tell yourself, "I didn't cheat. I simply made a not-so-great choice, and that is ok. I forgive myself, and I'm moving on."

Then, sit and *feel* the freedom. Words have the power to heal and the power to harm. We are choosing to use healing words and take back our power. Do you feel the *myself*-sized hole in your heart getting smaller?

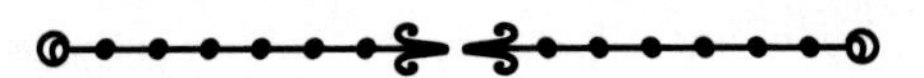

What's in your suitcase?

- Choice – great choice, good choice, not so great choice
- Megaphone (for louder cheering!)
- Tissues
- Full-length photo
- Album set up in your phone or on your computer where you will store your "becoming you" photos
- No Should Zone t-shirt and poster
- Your power
- Google maps
- Locks
- "Traffic Jam" written on an index card
- Print off the "Stay" card
- Book of positive affirmations
- Seasoning
- Forgiveness
- Choices
- Community
- Stop
- Idea about your destination
- Plan for saboteurs
- Plan for food pushers
- Trash bags
- Oxygen mask
- *WHY*

- Friedrich Nietzsche quote
- Photo of you
- Index cards
- Stake
- Hammer
- website
- Snap a photo – post it to the You Can't Eat Love Facebook page
- Join the private You Can't Eat Love Facebook group
- Workbook
- *So, I said to myself...*Journal
- Pens
- Highlighters

Life Hacks

- On this journey, we want to surround ourselves with thoughts and words that encourage us, especially when we hit a traffic jam. "Cheat" and "willpower" are not helpful. Maybe you can think of a few more. Write them down and throw them out of the window too!

Jackie says

- Put yourself first
- Learn to foam roll and stretch (YouTube has great videos)

Weblinks

https://linktr.ee/youcanteatlove

CHAPTER 10

Trigger Is Not Just The Name Of Roy Rogers' Horse

Just because no one else can heal or do your inner work for you doesn't mean you can, should, or need to do it alone.

Lisa Olivera

I remember people tossing around this term "trigger." I was absolutely certain they were confused. The only triggers I could think of were those on a gun or something that caused a bad person to do bad things. I did not understand how the word applied to me and eating until I cooked a brisket shortly after I started this journey.

I had cooked brisket many times over the years but never had an experience quite like this before. I went through a real-life example of "trigger." I will never forget it. Maybe this happened because I was starting to listen to me and myself when they talked to me.

On this particular day, most of my family was at the house for dinner. I pulled the brisket out of the oven, and as soon as the smell hit my nose, I was transported back to my grandmother's house. I could see Willie Mae taking the brisket out of the oven. The smell filled the kitchen, along with the smells of green rice (rice with spinach and beef consommé soup), green beans, freshly baked homemade biscuits dripping with melted butter, and chocolate merengue pie (yes, the exact same pie I mentioned at the start of this journey). I could hear my parents, my grandparents, aunts, uncles, siblings, and cousins outside. They were laughing and talking about how great dinner smelled.

Caught up in the moment I was remembering, I took the knife out of the drawer, sliced off some of the fat, and quickly ate it. I did it again and again. I realized what I was doing, but I did not want to lose the moment. Finally, I made myself stop. I sliced the brisket, served the plates, sat down, and enjoyed the meal with my family.

Since it is just the two of us, I will tell you a secret. If other people had not been at the house and looking forward to eating, I would have eaten as much of that brisket as I could. I would have been ashamed of myself later, but in the moment, I would have been "home" again. In that moment, I would have been back in happy times with people who had died years before.

When the memory of the family gathering at my grandmother's house came back to me, I finally understood how an event or food can "trigger" mindless eating. I realized my brain has a lot of cherished memories stored in different file cabinets. When I see, hear, or smell something that is like a keyword search on Google, the corresponding drawer flies open, holding all my memories. I want to hang on to the moment I am remembering as if it was occurring right now.

Remember we talked about how powerful our mind is? This is part of the power. Our mind wants us to be happy, and when those senses "trigger" a memory, our mind pulls out all the stops to make it as real as it was when it first happened.
How do we stay in the memory? By doing whatever it was that caused the drawer to open. For me in this case, that was eating the brisket and savoring the taste and the smell.

A note on sugar
I am not a scientist or nutritionist, but I will tell you my observation about another food: sugar. When I eat

refined sugar (which shows up in all kinds of crazy places like ketchup), I find myself hunting for something to eat. I have noticed if I avoid refined sugar, I do not feel as much of an urge to eat unplanned food.

My "tried all kinds of things before I found something that works" solution to the eating urge triggered by sugar is to grab protein. For you, maybe a walk or change of scenery will stop the hunt. You must discover what works for you. The best way to do this is to *be aware* of what you are thinking and feeling when you eat or even just see certain foods.

Celebrate good times--come on!

Holidays, celebrations, and parties can also be a danger zone. This is especially true if we do not pay attention to me and myself. Remember, all they are trying to do is protect you.

Honestly, I do not like Christmas or my birthday. It has nothing to do with the holiday or event itself. My dislike is related to the sad memories I have of my mother dying and when she passed away just three weeks before my birthday.

On this journey, I have been facing the overwhelming sadness of losing my mother along with regret. It has been hard. I have shed lots of tears and made lots of not-so-great choices. I have used my "drug of choice" to numb feelings I did not want to face. There have been lots of half-eaten half-gallons of Blue Bell ice cream.

But I am still standing. I did not let my "drug of choice" take over and cover up the pain. I stopped myself. I forgave myself. I told myself, "I understand." (Empathy is our friend.)

My last birthday and the recent holidays have not been as painful. I felt a little sad. I told me and myself I felt sad and it was ok. I did not need me and myself to protect me. I did not need "my drug of choice."

Learning to live with the memories and understanding how certain smells can take me and myself back has been a lot of work on my journey. I cannot tell you how many times me and myself wanted to park my car, get out, and walk home because they did not think it was worth it. That is when I stepped in and reminded me and myself *why* I was on this journey.

My *myself*-sized hole is getting smaller. I am enough. I am staying in the car.

Your *myself*-sized hole is getting smaller too. You are enough—and you are worth it. Your ***WHY*** is what will help you stay in your car and keep creeping forward when all you want to do is get out and walk home.

In your workbook, list your triggers and the holidays/celebrations that make you the most anxious (e.g., smells, sights, sounds, people, etc.). We will practice some strategies to keep them under control.

Strategy:

- → Name what you are feeling. It may be more than one thing, dig down and name all of the feelings
- → Acknowledge – "of course I feel....."
- → If it is a happy memory – savor the moment, sit quietly and reflect on it, then thank yourself for reminding you of it.
- → If it is not a happy memory – let your BFFITWWW comfort you and tell you "of

course you feel..." It is ok to cry. Stay with the memory as long as you can, hug yourself.

→ If it is an unhelpful memory, a memory about something you regret – forgive yourself, listen to yourself, and let your BFFITWWW comfort you. Talk out what you might do differently next time.

Always keep in mind, you are never alone.
Reach out.

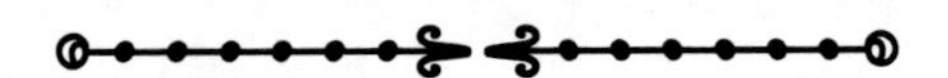

What's in your suitcase?

- More tissues
- Magnifying glass and binoculars to help spot triggers
- Choice – great choice, good choice, not so great choice
- Megaphone (for louder cheering!)
- Tissues
- Full-length photo
- Album set up in your phone or on your computer where you will store your "becoming you" photos
- No Should Zone t-shirt and poster
- Your power
- Google maps
- Locks
- "Traffic Jam" written on an index card
- Print off the "Stay" card
- Book of positive affirmations
- Seasoning
- Forgiveness
- Choices
- Community
- Stop
- Idea about your destination
- Plan for saboteurs

- Plan for food pushers
- Trash bags
- Oxygen mask
- ***WHY***
- Friedrich Nietzsche quote
- Photo of you
- Index cards
- Stake
- Hammer
- website
- Snap a photo – post it to the You Can't Eat Love Facebook page
- Join the private You Can't Eat Love Facebook group
- Workbook
- *So, I said to myself...*Journal
- Pens
- Highlighters

Life Hacks

- One of the hardest sentences I had to learn to say was "I feel...". Then I ask myself "why am I feeling....?" As I got more practice saying this, the easier it was to recognize the triggers and ask myself why I was being "triggered". If switching my thought process, distracting myself, or taking a short walk does not stop the "trigger", I will grab something high in protein – a protein drink (1st Phorm chocolate milkshake is my favorite), or a spoon full of peanut butter. The trick about peanut butter is I must close the jar and put it away before I eat the spoonful. I speak kindly to myself just as I would my very best friend in the whole wide world. (Don't ask me why, I just know that something high in protein stops the cravings from triggers faster than anything else I have tried. For me, the whole distraction thing becomes a fight of wills. And guess what wins.)

Jackie says

- Don't compare yourself to others
- Make sure you have a rest day

Weblinks

https://linktr.ee/youcanteatlove

SECTION III

Peeling Back the Layers

Motivation is like food for the brain.
You cannot get enough in one sitting.
It needs continual and regular top ups.
Peter Davies

CHAPTER 11

How Do We Get from Here to There?

Concentrate all of your thoughts upon the work at hand.
The sun's rays do not burn until brought into focus.
Alexander Graham Bell

Are you ready to get down to the nuts and bolts of this journey? Get ready to add even more things to your suitcase. We will be picking them up along the way.

Plans...it all starts with a plan

Choose the plan you will use to help you learn about food choices, portions, and calories. A lot of good options exist, including phone apps. I selected Weight Watchers. I still follow this framework, even now, years after reaching the weight that is manageable for me.

Select the plan that is easy for *you* to follow. Remember, this is *your* journey. You are behind the wheel. (If you haven't checked your calorie requirements yet, do it now! info.youcanteatlove.com)

Look around and see what will work for you. The two main principles to keep in mind when you are looking for a plan are 1.) Will it teach you what a balanced food plan looks like? and 2.) Is the weight-loss setting between 500-700 calories less than you normally consume?

The workbook contains a section where you can write down the pros and cons of different plans. This will help you make the best choice for *you*. If you have questions, reach out.

No matter which option you choose, I suggest you commit to writing down your food choices for the first six months of your journey. I know. I can hear you telling me all about the clicking, swiping, and scanning you can do. You can still click, swipe, and scan; just write down your food choices too.

> You can get downloadable pages from the Fit and Food Journal at http://youcanteatlove.com/journal . There is also a link to order the journal.

Trust me. I learned it is so much easier to be honest with myself when my food choices were there in black and white (or teal and white or pink and white; you get the idea). Our brains must learn this new relationship with food too. Writing activates a different part of your brain than clicking and swiping. I promise the six months will fly by.

Writing down your food choices also benefits you on those days when you make a not-so-great choice. You have a place from which you can have a conversation with yourself. Talk kindly to yourself about what was going on.

Then, you can practice making a different choice the next time. And yes, I do suggest practicing. Let us think about this for just a moment. Athletes, actors, musicians, and a lot of other people practice before they perform. Why? When it is time to perform, the ruts already exist, making it much easier to stay on the right track.

I am not telling you that practice will keep you from making not-so-good choices. I am telling you that practice will help you be aware, so you can make a better choice than you might have if you had not practiced.

(Sometimes I laugh when I think about my boys going through all my food journals. They will have written confirmation that their mother was operating from a different solar system. ☺)

There is no substitute for...well, yes, there is!

I am certain you have several recipes you and your family like to prepare to eat. I do too. One of the tricks I learned early in my journey is to be brave and experiment with substituting ingredients. Sometimes it worked out, and other times, well, we won't discuss those here. (We can talk about them later. Maybe over a cup of coffee with frothed ultra-filtered non-fat milk ☺).

As you consider what you might cook, look at the items high in fat and sugar and ask yourself, can I use something else? The whole substituting flour thing to reduce carbohydrates does not work out very well. Trust me. But some fats are better than other fats, and you can swap those. There is space in your workbook to brainstorm substitutions.

One of the first things I figured out was how to reduce the fat I used in cooking. Instead of putting oil in the pan, I would lightly spray olive oil directly onto the meat after patting the meat dry with a paper towel. (Let's put one of those refillable sprayers into our suitcase.) I would spread the oil evenly over the meat, add seasoning, and then put the meat into the hot skillet. This not only reduced the amount of fat I used in my cooking, but it also cut down on spatter and added great flavor to the meat.

Another one of my favorite swaps for fat early in my journey was no-fat cream cheese. You know the gravy you make after you fry pork chops? Yes, that gravy. After I cooked all the meat, I would lower the temperature just a bit, and then, I would add about an eighth of the non-fat cream cheese to the skillet along with two to four tablespoons of milk. (I also switched to ultra-filtered, non-fat milk, which is higher in protein and has zero sugar). Slowly, the cream cheese would melt into the milk. I added seasoning and served the pork chops. My husband never knew the difference. I will warn you the cream cheese does have a smidge of a sharp taste to it, but in my humble opinion, it tastes good.

My other favorite substitution is non-fat Greek yogurt for all things sour cream. I even use it to make buttermilk. (Just mix part yogurt and part milk, or Google it for more details.) I even swap out sour cream for non-fat Greek yogurt when we have tacos and baked potatoes. The added bonus is my family and I are getting more protein, which is also a great way to satisfy hunger.

A couple of other easy substitutions I use are non-fat half and half and fat-free evaporated milk. I make flan with the non-fat half and half, and my husband does not even notice a difference. The fat-free evaporated milk is a great way to take calories out of pumpkin pie.

I have listed some of my favorite substitutions in the workbook. There is room for you to add yours. Please share them on Facebook as well. I would like to know how you use substitutions.

Google search and I have become very good friends as I scour the internet, looking for ways to reduce the "not-so-good calories" for the food I am fixing. I have been very surprised by the suggestions and even more pleasantly surprised by the taste. Yes, you can have lower-calorie, healthier food that tastes good.

I am not going to suggest you eat *anything* that does not taste good. I have thrown out a lot of experiments. (Confession time again. I do not substitute brown sugar, honey, or sugar. I may reduce the amount I am using, but I do not use substitutions because of that whole tastes good thing. You do you.)

I am not on a diet. This is *my* lifestyle, and nowhere in the rules does it say I have to eat something that does not taste good. (I knew there had to be a perk to being an adult. ☺)

Now I'm a chef!
Before I started on this journey, my kitchen and I did not have a good relationship. In fact, when I was growing up, my dream job was to be a buyer for a clothing company. I would live in an apartment in downtown New York. I would eat out all the time and use my oven for book storage. I still hold onto parts of that dream, but I quit dreaming of using my oven as book storage. "Why?" I learned if I wanted to enjoy what I was eating, I had to learn to prepare it.

I know, I know. You don't want to go on a journey and have to be cooking all the time. I didn't either, *and* I still don't.

I found a current quality cookbook. I started preparing my meals from the recipes in the cookbook. My go-to cookbooks are from America's Test Kitchen. My number one choice is ***One Pan Wonders***.

I learned flavor is one of the main components of satisfying food. (The junk food/fast food people stumbled onto this secret a long time ago.) I realized higher quality food tastes better and satisfies me more quickly. I also learned that seasoning adds great flavor. (Did you know there is a whole world of seasoning beyond salt, pepper, garlic powder, and onion powder?)

Instead of fixing individual things every night, I would double the recipe and then portion at least half of it into freezer containers which I then labeled and stored in the freezer. Later, all I had to do was thaw the contents, dump them into a pot, add a smidge of water, cover the pot, and gently reheat the food while I prepared a salad or other side dish. This is great when I am in a hurry, tired, or just not inspired to cook.

If cooking is absolutely ***not*** your thing, or you don't have time to cook, that is ok. Lots of grocery stores now have fresh options that are easy to microwave. After microwaving, you can transfer the food to a real plate and feel as if you are eating a homemade dish. (No judgment on the not cooking thing. I am the one who wanted to use my oven for book storage.)

Remember, you are the only you in the world, and you are learning to treat you with kindness and caring. So, treat yourself to a couple of "make-your-life-easier" cooking tools. You are worth it, and you will be more inspired to cook. Three of my favorites are an air fryer, a smaller food processor, and the pineapple cutter/corer.

Also, let mealtime be a time to enjoy your BFF fixing a lovely meal for you. Set the table, get out your best dishes, and transfer those homemade or heat-and-eat meals onto that lovely plate. Experience and savor your food. As you get comfortable with new flavors, you will want to slowly enjoy them.

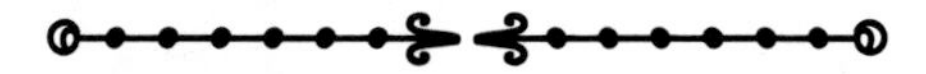

What's in your suitcase?

- Food plan/app
- Tracker – Fit and Food Journal
- Refillable oil sprayers for olive oil and regular oil

(I prefer *Misto* brand)
- Food storage containers (my personal preference is the *Rubbermaid Freshworks Produce Saver* – they work. Initial expense but you recover that in saved produce costs)
- More tissues
- Magnifying glass and binoculars to help spot triggers
- Choice – great choice, good choice, not so great choice
- Megaphone (for louder cheering!)
- Tissues
- Full-length photo
- Album set up in your phone or on your computer where you will store your "becoming you" photos
- No Should Zone t-shirt and poster
- Your power
- Google maps
- Locks
- "Traffic Jam" written on an index card
- Print off the "Stay" card
- Book of positive affirmations
- Seasoning
- Forgiveness
- Choices
- Community
- Stop
- Idea about your destination
- Plan for saboteurs
- Plan for food pushers
- Trash bags
- Oxygen mask
- ***WHY***
- Friedrich Nietzsche quote
- Photo of you
- Index cards
- Stake
- Hammer
- website
- Snap a photo – post it to the You

Can't Eat Love Facebook page
- Join the private You Can't Eat Love Facebook group
- Workbook
- *So, I said to myself...*Journal
- Pens
- Highlighters

Life Hacks

- Writing activates a different part of your brain and we are teaching our brain new tricks and habits
- I learned to cut out oil when sauteing onions, bell peppers, mushrooms, and other veggies. I put them in the skillet and add 2-4 Tbsps. of water, (the water will begin cooking the veggies) stir occasionally. The veggies will release their liquid. Cook until no liquid remains in the skillet, proceed with your recipe.
- When the recipe calls for browning meat in oil, pat the meat dry, spray with oil, season, rub all over the meat then put it into the hot pan (non-stick skillets don't brown as well as regular pans)
- Buttermilk substitute – ¾ cup yogurt mixed with ¼ cup milk (I use non-fat Greek yogurt and ultra-filtered milk because there is no fat and I get extra protein.)
- Pineapple cutter/corer (I use this at least once a week)
- I still weigh and measure everything. My scale is where I can grab it easily. Comes in very handy for baking. Don't guess – weigh and measure.
- Air fryer
- Small food processor
- Slow cooker or Instapot

Jackie Says

- Track your food. If your nutrition is not right, you will not reach your goal
- Prioritize protein

Weblinks

https://linktr.ee/youcanteatlove

CHAPTER 12

Greens, Greens, And More Greens

He does not know his own strength who has not met adversity.

William Samuel Johnson

The pantry is bare

Have you ever heard people say, "To eat healthily, shop the perimeter of the grocery store and stay away from the middle as much as possible"? I have, but I did not understand what they (There are those "they" people again. I am going to make it a bucket list item to meet them!) were talking about until I started changing what I was eating. All the great choices are on the perimeter of the store unless you go to one of those stores that hide the yogurt in the middle with the ice cream. So, I had to change how I shopped.

Before I began this journey, I would go to the store with only a few ideas of what I wanted to have for dinners and lunches. I rarely had a real plan. I had an idea of what proteins I wanted to fix and kind of knew what I wanted to go with the protein. So, a lot of times, I had to make several trips to the store in between my major shopping.

While in the store, I would grab a tiny amount of fresh fruits and vegetables and some proteins. Then, I would spend most of my time going up and down the aisles, picking up items I thought would be good to have on hand. I reached for easy over yummy, so most of the meals were not very satisfying.

Now, I sit down with a pen and paper to create my menu. I write down ideas for 10-15 main dishes, leaving a few lines in between ideas. Then, I go back and write down ideas for side dishes. I do a quick check of items I have on hand and make a note of items I will need. I pull out cookbooks and quickly look for recipes. I list any ingredients I need under the main dishes to make it easy for me to sort ingredients. I want to make sure I don't end up with twelve cans of tomato paste and no tomato sauce.

> You can download sample menus, menu planner sheets, sample grocery lists, and blank grocery lists on the website http://youcanteatlove.com/menu

Next, I start making my grocery list. It helps me to decide what meals I will prepare within the first seven days. I highlight on my list the fresh ingredients and bulk items I will need for the last seven to ten days. I also highlight what items I need to buy more than one of such as cartons of eggs and yogurt.

> *Do you have just a moment? I can be honest with you, can't I? Let's stop and think about this. First, we spend time deciding what we need to buy. Then, we make a list. There is travel time to the store, time in the store picking up everything on our list, and travel time back home. And then, we must put everything away (I appreciate the sackers asking if I need help to my car, but where we all need help is when we get home.) How much time is that? And we have not even started cooking yet! Now, do you see why I thought books should be stored in the oven?*

I try to limit my trips to the grocery store to about every two to three weeks. Why? Going to the store less means there is less chance for food that does not know how to behave ending up in my house.

A trick to help me get by on fewer trips to the store is to purchase a lot of items via online ordering. My grocery store offers free pickup if I schedule future pickups (more than 4 days out). I create an order to be picked up early in the morning about seven days out from my "in-person" shopping trip. I order all the highlighted items on my list, marking them off as I go. I know to get the remaining items on my list when I go to the store. This task takes me about twenty minutes, but it makes my life easier in the long run. If you are very busy, I strongly encourage you to use a store pickup service to save yourself time, reduce frustration, and especially keep from paying for items that just jumped into your cart.

Since beginning this journey, I rarely buy boxed foods—but that is a personal choice. You do *you*. Just know that not all boxed foods are created equally. Read the labels and look for hidden sugar. Choose flavor and satisfaction over quantity and simplicity. Trust me; flavor will win over quantity in the satisfaction game. And yes, I know the more satisfying options sometimes cost more, but you *will* save in the long run.

Post your menu on the refrigerator so you can easily remember your game plan. I create my menu in an Excel spreadsheet. I print it out, put it in a sheet protector, and hang it on the freezer door along with a dry erase pen. As I prepare each meal, I mark it off the list.

Another trick that helps me is to write the days of the week next to the meal options on my menu. That gives me one less thing to worry about when my schedule is crazy. I know what meals I will prepare each day.

Waste it or waist it

Can I tell you a secret? (I do seem to be telling you a lot of those. I hope you don't mind ❤) I throw perfectly good food away. I know, "horrors" as my mother would say. Let me tell you a story to explain why I throw perfectly good food away.

When my two older boys were little, I put one of them in time-out for something he did. (Time-out was the school of thought back then.) This resulted in me getting frustrated over having to constantly monitor the time-out. Nobody learned anything other than to get more upset. Maybe I did not do the time-out "correctly," according to the time-out police, but, for me, it did not work.

After that, I would put items instead of my boys in time-out. If there was a loud discussion over a toy, game, puzzle, or anything else, I would tell the boys, "It seems the cars are having a hard time following the rules today. I am going to put them in time-out until they learn how to follow the rules." I would place the offending item on a high shelf and leave it there for about an hour.

In the meanwhile, peace would fall over the house again. The kids would calm down and forget about the squabble. I would not get upset.

Putting items in time-out had another benefit besides me keeping my tiny sliver of sanity. I taught my children (in a backward way) that if something does not follow the rules, there will be a consequence. Since I focused on the behavior/actions and not the people, there was no shaming and blaming.

Now, what does this have to do with food? There are certain foods in my house that do not know how to behave. Like the cookie dough we talked about much earlier. And let's not forget about the chocolate cheesecake. Chocolate candy, cookies, and ice cream all have a very bad scorecard in my house. I have found it is much better to throw them away than to fight with them because they usually win. Maybe not today, but someday soon, they will win.

So, here comes that useless word *willpower*. We talked about willpower briefly in Chapter 7. Will power is another word for "fighting to delay gratification."

Since chocolate is like that bad boyfriend my parents did not want me to date, I am not likely to delay any kind of gratification. Nope, it's not happening. I have accepted chocolate and I cannot peacefully exist in the same house. *And that is ok*. I *can* peacefully exist with a lot of other foods.

Does this mean I never have chocolate in the house? No. My husband will bring chocolate into the house, and I will tolerate it for as long as I can. Then, I will throw it away—sometimes after I have sneakily eaten about half of it—and tell him I don't know what happened to it. See, this is a journey.

What food is *your* kryptonite? In your workbook, make your list of foods that don't know how to behave. Then, we can work on a plan of action. Remember, we are learning to not lie to me and myself. We are also learning to be kind to ourselves, and willpower is anything but kind. We all need as much kindness and grace as possible on this journey.

Why set yourself up to not be successful? (We will talk about that word fail in just a moment.) Set yourself up to succeed. Set yourself up to have kind, encouraging thoughts about your relationship with food. The more we play the shame and blame game, the deeper those ruts get and the harder it is to drive in the new ruts. Our goal is to make our life easier and lighter so we when we do hit a traffic jam (e.g., a misbehaving food comes into the house), we stay in the car instead of parking it and walking home.

If you are struggling to avoid a food, throw it away. You can waste it or waist it. Which one is going to be more expensive? Toss the food and walk away, telling yourself how proud you are of yourself. *You* are in control and not the food. Then, keep moving forward.

You've got this. Give yourself a giant cheer and throw in a hug from me. It sure would be nice to have a heart emoji right about now. 😊

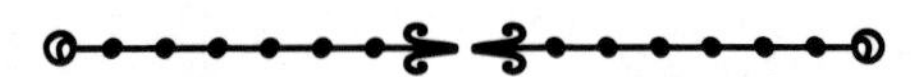

What's in your suitcase?

- Bigger megaphone
- Menu plan
- Grocery list
- More trash bags
- Hug from me
- Food plan/app
- Tracker – Fit and Food Journal
- Refillable oil sprayers for olive oil and regular oil (I prefer *Misto* brand)
- Food storage containers (my personal preference is the *Rubbermaid Freshworks Produce Saver* – they do work. Initial expense but you recover that in saved produce costs)
- More tissues
- Magnifying glass and binoculars to help spot triggers
- Choice – great choice, good choice, not so great choice
- Megaphone (for louder cheering!)
- Tissues
- Full-length photo

- Album set up in your phone or on your computer where you will store your "becoming you" photos
- No Should Zone t-shirt and poster
- Your power
- Google maps
- Locks
- "Traffic Jam" written on an index card
- Print off the "Stay" card
- Book of positive affirmations
- Seasoning
- Forgiveness
- Choices
- Community
- Stop
- Idea about your destination
- Plan for saboteurs
- Plan for food pushers
- Trash bags
- Oxygen mask
- ***WHY***
- Friedrich Nietzsche quote
- Photo of you
- Index cards
- Stake
- Hammer
- website
- Snap a photo – post it to the You Can't Eat Love Facebook page
- Join the private You Can't Eat Love Facebook group
- Workbook
- *So, I said to myself...*Journal
- Pens
- Highlighters

Life Hacks

- Shop the perimeter of the store
- Place a pick-up order about 5-7 days out from your grocery shopping day
- Homemade pasta (higher in protein and tastes so much better than store-bought) 10 ounces of flour

and 3 room-temperature LARGE (not extra-large) eggs. I make mine in the food processor. (Flour in first, pulse about 5 times, then add eggs and process until it starts sticking together. Remove from processor and knead until smooth, wrap in plastic wrap and let it sit, continue as with handmade.) It can be made by pouring the flour into a mound on a cutting surface (I am lazy so I will do it on parchment paper or some type of cling wrap), make a well in the middle, lightly scramble the eggs, pour into the well. Using a knife or chopstick start pulling the flour in and mixing it with the egg. After you have pulled all of the flour in, knead the dough until it feels smooth. Wrap in plastic wrap and let it sit for at least 30 minutes. Then you can cut into 4-5 pieces, roll each piece out, then cut each section into strips one at a time. Boil in well-salted water for about 2.5-3 minutes, drain and toss with about 1-2T of olive oil or other seasonings, add protein and serve.

- **FAIL** – Rethink what you hear. Now, I want you to hear First Attempt In Learning. Give yourself grace and kindness. FAIL is now shorthand and a signal to you that it is a First Attempt In Learning, tomorrow or next time will be better. You never truly fail (see the difference in how the word is written?) until you quit. Don't quit. I believe in you.

Jackie says

- Master fundamental moves like squats and lunge

Weblinks

https://linktr.ee/youcanteatlove

CHAPTER 13

To Move Or Not To Move - That Is The Question

The gem cannot be polished without friction nor man perfected without trials.

Chinese Proverb

Exercise. I counted that as a four-letter word I tried to avoid saying, much less doing. Oh. My. Gosh. I do not like being hot. I hate to sweat. I hate to breathe hard.

As you continue this journey, be careful about what words you consider to be four-letter words. You may have to do some backtracking. I did.

Aren't steps those things I don't climb?

I still remember attending a meeting and hearing some of the people there bragging about their fit watches. (I had heard of these watches but did not pay much attention to them since the only thing I was interested in measuring was my food.) These people were probably in their 70's and getting more than 8,000 steps a day. Can you believe that? I **knew** I was getting at *least* 20,000 steps in a day. (We will not discuss my age. I believe age is a matter of perspective anyway. Just suffice to say, I did not consider myself as old as these people were.)

So, knowing how *much* younger *and* fitter I was, I decided to track my steps and see how far over 20,000 I went. My phone had a health app on it. I turned on the app and went about my day. Imagine my horror when I looked at the app and saw proof of my struggle to even get close to 2,000 steps in one day. And I thought I was running laps around the "old"' people at the meeting. (Seriously, typewriter people, you need to add smack my head emojis to the keyboard.)

I must confess (I seem to be doing a lot of confessing here, hope you don't mind 😉) I thought maybe there was a glitch in the app, so I checked again over the next several days. Nope. No glitch. ☹ I was only getting about 2,000 – 3,000 steps a day.

What did I do next? I did what I am going to suggest to you if you hate sweating and being hot as much as I did. I got *super* inefficient. I know you are trying to figure out what the heck that has to do with steps. Here are just a few things I became inefficient in:

- Unloading the dryer. (I started unloading the dryer in three to four loads instead of one or two.)
- Carrying folded laundry to be put away. (I carried the individual stacks of folded laundry one at a time.)
- Parking my car. (I parked my car at the back of the parking lot, which had the added bonus of no nicks or dings.)
- Carrying groceries. (I carried fewer bags of groceries at a time when unloading the car.)

> Your workbook has this information in it and some space for you to write your own ideas

Do you see what I was doing? I broke down ordinary tasks, so I could trick myself into taking more steps. Remember that whole mind thing and how we can tell it stories? Here is a perfect example. I tricked myself.
As I took more steps during the day, the week, and the month, I gained confidence in myself. I could feel myself moving better. I could actually walk somewhere. Plus, the extra weight was coming off a bit quicker. (Still hated to sweat or be hot.) I also gained confidence in how I looked.

I wanted to know how far I was walking. I bought a fitness watch so I could get a more accurate count of my steps. (We will talk about the watch more in just a bit.) I started by setting a timer for five minutes and walking in a circle in my backyard during that time. I can hear you saying to yourself, "That is not very long." You are correct, *but* it was a lot longer than I had been walking. My goal was to walk at least 250 steps every hour.

Remember, we are driving a new car down a muddy road to make new ruts. When we begin a journey, it is not like a video game where we can get a power-up and skip ahead several moves. We must travel each and every single mile, no matter how fast or slowly we cover the ground.

Why am I telling you this? Because I want to remind you to be kind to yourself. Meet yourself where you are and not where you or someone else imagines you *should* be. (Let's get that *should* word out of our vocabulary.)

> *There is absolutely nothing wrong with where you are. It just is. It just is where you are. You are also on a journey heading for somewhere else. And that is ok.*

As each week came and went, I would add a few more minutes to my walking until I was up to ten minutes. (Celebration!) My walking created a path in the backyard—very much like the new ruts I was trying to create in my mind.

Next, I would walk down the street and add time to my goal. I found it easier to move. I went farther and still had energy when I got back home. My knees and hips hurt less. Getting out and walking became fun. I looked forward to the alarm I had set to ring to remind me it was time to walk.

Think about how long you *know* you can walk and where you can walk. Write this down in your workbook. Make a date with yourself and set a reminder on your phone to walk. You are taking care of you. Celebrate that! Share with us on Facebook so we can celebrate with you too.

Check your phone to see if it has a fitness app on it. If it does, turn the app on and start checking your steps. Set a timer for a length of time you *know* you can walk. Turn on some tunes and walk.

Each week add a minute to your walking time (or however many minutes you *know* you can add and not feel defeated). Little by little, you are moving and getting to know yourself a bit more. Buy a pair of rubber boots (that make you smile when you look at them) and a good raincoat so you can walk even in rainy weather. (Tip: Wear a hat under the hood of your raincoat to keep the hood from collapsing onto your face.) I prefer a raincoat over an umbrella because I like to have my arms free and burn more calories. As with everything else, you do you. That is most important.

Wait—there's more!

If you are like me, you will reach a point where just walking feels a bit dull. You will probably start looking for some other exercises to add to your routine. Remember to *meet you where you are*.

I began with simple exercises that challenged most of my muscles. And before you ask if running was one of them, the answer is "Nope, nope, nope." I do not run. I have tried all kinds of ways to trick myself, and the old me keeps kicking the new tricks out.

Now, I do not have anything against people who do run. I admire them. If you like to run, that is amazing. It is a great cardio exercise. I will wave as you go streaking by.

You can find lots of beginner routines by searching the internet. (If you are looking for a great resource to get you started, I recommend ***6-Minute Fitness at 60+: Simple Home Exercises to Reclaim Strength, Balance, and Energy in 15 Days*** by Jonathan Su with simple exercises to help you get started. Disregard the age reference in the title. This is a great book with explanations and routines to get you moving. I use the routine as part of my workouts.) Some of the fitness apps have exercise routines that are great for beginners too. Test them out.

Take your time and find something that appeals to you. Choose something that does not take a lot of time, fancy equipment, or space. If you are not strong enough *now*, that is ok. Now is all you are worried about. Tomorrow, now will be different. At this point, all you are trying to do is work some of your muscles so you can feel even more confident when you move. A bonus is your muscles will start toning and you will start occupying less space than you used to. (And yes, I still hated being hot and sweating.)

After you pick your exercises, decide how many days a week you are going to exercise and what time you are going to exercise. Like everything else we have talked about, meet you where you are. Do not schedule your exercise at five in the morning when you struggle to get out of bed before six. Do not schedule your exercise at five in the afternoon when you are running kids around to their activities. Set a number of days to exercise that is reasonable for *you*. For you, Saturday and Sunday may be the only days that may work. That is ok. You make the rules *for you*.

Make the time you choose to exercise sacred. Schedule this time on your calendar or wherever you keep track of your life. Create a reminder on your phone or on your computer.

In your workbook, write down your chosen exercises, how long you will exercise, and the days and times you will exercise. This is your exercise plan.

Lately, we haven't talked much about the oxygen mask you packed. Well, making a date with yourself and setting aside that time is part of putting on your own oxygen mask first. Scheduling time to exercise makes you just as important as the rest of the people in your life.

You must make you a priority because *no one else will*. **We teach people how to treat us.** When my husband would comment on my exercising, I would smile, nod, and keep going (because a lot of the time I had on my headphones and could not hear him. 😉)

Oxygen mask on. Commit to you. You do you.

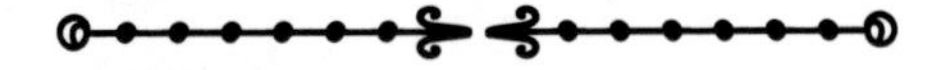

What's in your suitcase?

- Rubber boots
- Raincoat
- Exercises for beginners
- Health app or fitness tracker
- Timer (a lot of phones have a timer)
- Alarm set to remind to go out and walk

- Headphones/music or podcasts
- Bigger megaphone
- Menu plan
- Grocery list
- More trash bags
- Hug from me
- Food plan/app
- Tracker – Fit and Food Journal
- Refillable oil sprayers for olive oil and regular oil (I prefer *Misto* brand)
- Food storage containers (my personal preference is the *Rubbermaid Freshworks Produce Saver* – they work. Initial expense but you recover that in saved produce costs)
- More tissues
- Magnifying glass and binoculars to help spot triggers
- Choice – great choice, good choice, not so great choice
- Megaphone (for louder cheering!)
- Tissues
- Full-length photo
- Album set up in your phone or on your computer where you will store your "becoming you" photos
- No Should Zone t-shirt and poster
- Your power
- Google maps
- Locks
- "Traffic Jam" written on an index card
- Print off the "Stay" card
- Book of positive affirmations
- Seasoning
- Forgiveness
- Choices
- Community
- Stop
- Idea about your destination
- Plan for saboteurs

- Plan for food pushers
- Trash bags
- Oxygen mask
- ***WHY***
- Friedrich Nietzsche quote
- Photo of you
- Index cards
- Stake
- Hammer
- website
- Snap a photo – post it to the You Can't Eat Love Facebook page
- Join the private You Can't Eat Love Facebook group
- Workbook
- *So, I said to myself...*Journal
- Pens
- Highlighter

Life Hacks

- Being inefficient is a painless way to increase your activity
- Make appointments with yourself just like you do for any other activity in your life, Make the time sacred. Oxygen Mask – use it.
- Set a time for how long you are going to move and then add 1 minute each week.

Jackie says

- Invest in a great pair of shoes! (NoBull are my favorites)

Weblinks

https://linktr.ee/youcanteatlove

CHAPTER 14

I Do Not Want to be the Rock

Great things never came from comfort zones.
Anonymous

After I had been on this journey for about a year, I decided to join a gym. Why did I join a gym? Well, it all goes back to that very important question—***WHY.*** My gym why lines up with my big why.

I realized I believed in myself more than I had when I began this journey. I was ready to take myself to the next level, and for me, joining a gym was the best way to do that. A gym had the equipment I did not have. So, I could do more than I was doing at home.

What is more, I would see other people at the gym who were trying to be the best they could be. This inspired me. Gyms are not full of bodybuilders like The Rock; they are full of people just like you and me—people trying to live their best lives in the only body they have. Gyms are full of people putting on their oxygen masks first. (And I learned these people are too busy breathing and counting to care what I am doing, so I don't have to fear everyone looking at me.)

Are you ready to go to the next level? Could joining a gym be one way to do that for *you*? Think about your next level "gym" why and write it in your workbook. Does it line up with your big ***WHY***?

Joining a gym

May I tell you a secret about the process of joining a gym? You go to the gym and express your interest in joining. You will be introduced to a salesperson (usually not a trainer) who will show you around the gym. Their job is to get you to sign up before you walk out. Most gyms have guest passes for a few days or a week.

Google the gyms in your area. See if they offer guest passes, and if they do, take advantage of them. Try out the gyms in your area, not once or even twice, but for all. the days allotted. Go at the times you would usually exercise.

Notice things while you try out the various gyms. How many people are there? Do you have to wait for the equipment? How comfortable are you there? Different gyms have different "vibes" or energy. How comfortable you feel at a gym is important. You will be paying for the privilege to sweat in the space, so you want to make the best choice possible.

Think of these scouting missions as dates. You can date more than one person and you can go on more than one date with one person. This does not mean you are in a long-term relationship. You are only dating. Enjoy the experience and then decide which one you want to "spend the rest of your life with."

> In the workbook, you can keep track of the gyms in your area, the pass policy, and your experience. This will help you make your decision.

Ok, so, you are finished dating and now you are ready to commit. You have done your homework and made your decision. Remember, the first person you meet at the gym is usually a salesperson. Let them do their thing. Let them answer any questions you thought of when you were dating. If they do not mention at least one free session with a trainer, bring it up. Tell them you are interested. You don't have to set up the session right away; you can set it up later.

Did I do all of this when I was looking for a gym? No. But I wish I would have.

Congratulations on going to the next level. Joining a gym is a great way to take care of yourself. Be sure to cheer loudly all the way home. Share on Facebook so we can all celebrate with you. Know that I am sending you lots of high tens.

Add your new gym membership to your suitcase. It fits right in there along with your oxygen mask, food plan, feelings, etc. I cannot wait to see what else we pick up.

I see you are getting the hang of putting on your oxygen mask first. Now, treat yourself to some good headphones so you can really enjoy your tunes while using all that exercise equipment.

Once you join the gym, adjust your exercise appointments and reminders accordingly. Make certain you allow for travel time. Nothing is worse than rushing and racing to get from one place to the other, especially if the other place is the gym. (Screen shot your appointment/reminder and post it on Facebook.)

Finding a trainer

During the first two or three weeks at the gym, look around and notice the trainers. Watch them with their clients. What kind of clients are they? If possible, listen to how the trainers talk to their clients. Does the client have their undivided attention (that is what you are paying for)? Or is the trainer looking around, talking to other people, or worse, on their phone.

When you get home, make notes about the trainers in your workbook. Also, do some research. Most gyms have a list of the trainers on their website along with a short bio on each trainer. Check out that information to help you narrow down your "targets. Mark off trainers that would not be a good fit for you. You usually have one "introductory" session, so you do not want to waste it on a bad fit.

After you think you have settled on one or two trainers, go to the friendly salesperson, and let them know you are ready to schedule your introductory session. Tell them which trainer(s) you would like. Usually, the trainer will contact you and set up the date and time. If you do not hear from someone within forty-eight hours, find a manager and let them know, so they can quickly take care of the issue. (The oxygen mask is handy, isn't it?)

After you have your initial appointment with the trainer, add it to your calendar. Post on Facebook so we can cheer you on. (Remember, celebrating helps us drive the car down the muddy road and make new ruts. The more celebrating, the deeper the ruts. 😊) I want you to be prepared for your time with the trainer. First, the trainer will ask you what your workout goals are. My gym goal was to get stronger, trim, and tone all over. Aren't you glad you are clear on your ***why***? You will be able to tell the trainer exactly what your goal is. When you finish the first session, the trainer will usually offer you more sessions at a reduced price.

Although you have already learned much about the trainer from your research and watching them, do not be afraid to ask questions. Ask the trainer about their background and training philosophy. Remember, this is someone you are hiring to help ***you*** on your journey, not the other way around.

This is your time. *Your money*. And *<u>your why</u>*. Oxygen mask.

Pay attention to how the trainer talks to you and how you feel as you work with them. Make sure they are meeting you where you are. A great trainer will evaluate your body, point out areas that need to be strengthened, and make some suggestions on how to do that.

One of the things that sold me on my trainer was she immediately recognized I had a problem with my knees. I never knew that. I only knew my knees did not line up right and certain exercises never looked like the pictures. She told me I needed to focus on strengthening my knees so training the rest of my body would be effective. (She was right, by the way.)

Training is a bit like baking. If you get one ingredient slightly off, you end up with a flat cake. All the more reason to choose your trainer wisely.

At the end of the first session, if you feel good and believe the trainer is a good fit for you, sign up for the introductory package. But let the trainer know you will be meeting with them only one time a week. Ask them for a copy of the workout so you can do it the other two to three days a week on your own.

Why do I suggest this? Let's think about it.

Remember, you are paying the trainer for the privilege to train you. Not the other way around. They will likely be watching and notice whether or not you come to the gym between sessions.

You are new to the gym scene. You are new to working out. You are just starting to have confidence in yourself and believe you can keep moving on this journey.

What you need right now is someone to demonstrate a series of exercises to you. You need someone to show you correct form, correct breathing, and correct progression. Then, you need to practice so your body gets used to this new thing.

If you have signed up for six training sessions, that means you are tricking yourself to be in the gym for at least six weeks. That's enough time to build a new habit. An added benefit is that you will likely see some changes in your shape and strength before the end of the six weeks. Like the old "sweat and reward" system, those changes will encourage you to keep going to the gym.

If after the introductory package, you don't have the resources to continue with a trainer, that is ok. You now have six different exercise routines you can do on your own. If you go to the gym three days a week, you still have two weeks' worth of exercises because you will do a different set each time you go. See, you *are* doing you!

I do suggest that you set aside some money to meet with a trainer for at least one session once a quarter. This will allow you to update your routine and keep up with the changes in your strength, stamina, and shrinking form.

In your workbook, write down your plan for your training and working out on your own. Mark off each workout as you do it. Give yourself a much-deserved cheer each time.

A game-changer

I must admit I played at going to the gym for quite a while. I didn't understand the machines or how to effectively train. I knew how to walk on the treadmill and ride the stationary bike. I looked at the graphics on the machines and tried my best to imitate them. I was doing something, but it was more like trying to clean a window with a dirty paper towel. I was not making much progress.

Then I met Jackie.

My youngest son suggested we join a new gym because they had more and better equipment than the gym where I was going. I did the introductory session and agreed to several more sessions. But I was not completely happy with the trainer with whom I was working. I couldn't put my finger on my dissatisfaction. It was just there.

Then, one day while I was training, the trainer told me she was moving and handing me off to someone else who would be calling me. Over a week passed. No call came.

So, I approached a trainer one morning in the gym and told her I had not heard from anyone. She was working with another trainer whom I had watched closely. I liked how the second trainer worked with her clients. This second trainer—Jackie—spoke up right away and said she would take my information, give me a call later in the morning, and get me set up to work with her.

The rest, as they say, is history. I have been working with Jackie for three years now. She helped me get the last twenty pounds off and totally reshaped my body. What she has done for my confidence is incredible.

Finding a trainer who encourages and believes in you gives you the confidence to push yourself when you don't think you can. I still don't like to sweat. I still believe breathing while sweating is overrated, but I LOVE how strong I have become.

I am not telling you to hire a trainer and keep paying them from now until the end of time. I am saying I decided to take care of myself and reach my goals. I have given up some things so I can work out with a trainer once a week.

Remember, you must meet you where you are and do *you*. It is *your* oxygen mask. Put it on, and then, take care of the other people.

All bull, no cows

Just like with anything you do in life; you must have the right equipment to get the job done correctly. I bought the dri-fit exercise pants, dri-fit shirts, socks, and "cute" tennis shoes. I looked like all the rest of the people in the gym.

At first, I didn't know I was missing something.

One day, my son was telling me about a pair of shoes he had bought for himself and what a difference they made in how he worked out. The shoes were designed for weight training. He felt more stable in them.

Since my biggest problem was my knees "falling in," I thought the shoes my son mentioned might help. The brand of the shoes was NoBull www.nobullproject.com. This company's shoes have very unique designs, colors, bottoms, and laces. I ordered my pair and waited for them to arrive. (They did cost more than I paid for other workout shoes, but they are worth every single penny.) I told Jackie I had ordered the shoes, and she was very curious to see what the "fuss" was about.

I still remember the first time I put my NoBull shoes on. I felt so much more stable.

And then, the big test came. Twenty lunges forward and then back. I immediately felt a difference in how my foot was planted on the ground. I immediately felt my knees stay lined up over my ankles where they were supposed to be. And, immediately, Jackie could see a huge difference in how I performed the exercises. She was sold. I was beyond sold. I could feel muscles I did not know I had.

Within a month of wearing my NoBulls, my legs began to change shape. The muscles started tightening and toning the way they were supposed to, and my knees got stronger. I could tell such a difference when I wore NoBull shoes, I bought a pair for everyday wear.

I wore my everyday NoBull shoes all over London. I walked well over 25,000 steps a day. I walked up and down stairs and on and off trains. I did lots of standing and never once did my legs, hips, knees, or feet hurt.

I have already worn out two pairs of NoBulls, and I am about to wear out a third pair. I highly recommend them especially to people just starting to work out. They will help you keep your feet in the correct position. I also recommend them for daily wear for the exact same reason.

Currently, I have five pairs of NoBull shoes. Jackie owns about six pairs. After seeing what a difference the NoBull shoes made for me, she started wearing them and recommending them to everyone. Before the gym shut down due to the COVID-19 pandemic, about forty people who went there switched to wearing NoBull shoes, and most of them had more than one pair.

Is there a birthday or other gift-giving occasion coming up? Shop the NoBull site and send suggestions to your friends and relatives. I cannot wait to hear about your experience with NoBull trainers. When you get yours, post a photo on Facebook, the NoBull Facebook page, and #youcanteatlove.

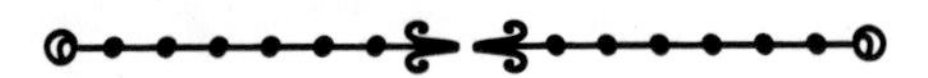

What's in your suitcase?

- Fanny pack or phone holder if you don't have cordless headphones
- Gym membership
- Date for Free Session
- Quality workout shoes
- Rubber boots
- Raincoat
- Exercises for beginners
- Health app or fitness tracker
- Timer (a lot of phones have a timer)
- Alarm set to remind to go out and walk
- Headphones/mus ic or podcasts
- Bigger megaphone
- Menu plan
- Grocery list
- More trash bags
- Hug from me
- Food plan/app
- Tracker – Fit and Food Journal
- Refillable oil sprayers for olive oil and regular oil (I prefer *Misto* brand)

- Food storage containers (my personal preference is the *Rubbermaid Freshworks Produce Saver* – they work. Initial expense but you recover that in saved produce costs)
- More tissues
- Magnifying glass and binoculars to help spot triggers
- Choice – great choice, good choice, not so great choice
- Megaphone (for louder cheering!)
- Tissues
- Full-length photo
- Album set up in your phone or on your computer where you will store your "becoming you" photos
- No Should Zone t-shirt and poster
- Your power
- Google maps
- Locks
- "Traffic Jam" written on an index card
- Print off the "Stay" card
- Book of positive affirmations
- Seasoning
- Forgiveness
- Choices
- Community
- Stop
- Idea about your destination
- Plan for saboteurs
- Plan for food pushers
- Trash bags
- Oxygen mask
- ***WHY***
- Friedrich Nietzsche quote
- Photo of you
- Index cards
- Stake
- Hammer
- website
- Snap a photo – post it to the You Can't Eat Love Facebook page

- Join the private You Can't Eat Love Facebook group
- Workbook
- *So, I said to myself...*Journal
- Pens
- Highlighters

Life Hacks

- You can explore a gym before joining
- Some gyms offer a discount/specials for people over a certain age
- Some insurance companies will cover a gym membership
- Set appointments/reminders for all activity including walks and the gym

Jackie says

- A good trainer is focused
- A good trainer asks you a lot of questions

Weblinks

https://linktr.ee/youcanteatlove

CHAPTER 15
There Is A Reason They Give Stars To Kindergartners

Every day of your life is a special occasion.
Thomas S. Morrison

Tricks and treats?
One of the best books I have ever read about behavior and rewards was ***Don't Shoot the Dog*** by Karen Pryor. I know, what in the heck does a book about shooting dogs have to do with me? Well, first, the book is not about shooting dogs. The book talks about how to reward to get the behavior you want and how to ignore to squash the behavior you do not want.

From reading the book, I learned the responsibility for the behavior falls on me, not my dog. A dog (or another trainable animal) is going to do what it is going to do. A dog will also keep doing whatever you give feedback on, regardless of what it is. For example, the dog starts barking at a passerby and you start yelling. Your yelling is the feedback that reinforced the barking. To stop or deter the barking, you must get the dog to focus on something else *and* reward the dog when it shifts its focus. (You might want to read the book after you finish this one.)

Now, let's move beyond a dog. Small children (and big ones too) operate from the same principle. Let's say you go to the store. You are planning on picking up a few items, and along the way, your child sees a coloring book they absolutely ***must*** have. So, you *know* what happens next. The child starts asking for the coloring book. (Actually, they tell you.)

The more times you say no, the louder the "request" gets until you are faced with a full-on temper tantrum in the middle of the store. Because everyone is staring at you and thinking, "What a terrible parent you are," you grab the coloring book and get out of the store as quickly as possible. Do you see what happened? You accidentally taught the child a temper tantrum was going to get them what they want. Just like yelling at the dog taught the dog to bark.

> *I must confess again. After I read* ***Don't Shoot the Dog****, I started looking at the people in my life and figured out how I could change some of their behavior using the principles in the book. Yes, it even works on my husband, but don't tell him.* 😉

Now, let's get back to changing our behavior with food. You are trying to drive new ruts in your brain. Our brains like to be rewarded. They like to feel happy. They want more of whatever makes them happy. So, what can you do to make your brain happy?

I will share what I did. I went to McDonald's around lunchtime and was determined to not get my usual order of a Big Mac, large fries, and a large Diet Coke (with no ice). I was only going to order a large Diet Coke with no ice. So, I pulled up to the speaker and quickly (before I could change my mind) ordered a large Diet Coke with no ice and said, "That's all." I paid at the window and picked up my drink. Then, I drove forward a bit, braked the car, took my hands off the steering wheel, and shouted as loudly as I could, "YES, YES, YES! I did it!"

True story. And boy, did that feel good. Yes, I was concerned about people thinking I was crazy, but then I realized what they thought was not as important as my journey (oxygen mask). This is what I do over and over again when I choose a good or great choice over a "hard-to-turn-down," not-so-good choice. Depending on where I am, I will either cheer silently or wait until I am alone and can enjoy a very loud cheer.

We are all on a journey, right? Some of us are on journeys to improve our lives. We are learning new ways to live. Think about how you feel when your family or good friends cheer you on or celebrate with you. Think about how happy your brain feels and how much you look forward to the next time.

Now, I understand your family and friends are not always with you. But guess who is? *You are always with you.* Become your very best cheerleader. Get loud and celebrate when you make tough great choices and even good choices. Forgive yourself for the not-so-great choices. In your workbook, list some of the choices you would like to change and how you will celebrate the change.

Stars, stars and so many more stars

I often remind people we give stars to kindergartners for a reason. It is the exact same reason we give a dog a treat when they do what we want them to do. We want them to repeat the behavior.

So, start giving yourself some stars. If you are a visual person, create a chart you put someplace where only you can see it. On your chart, list behaviors you want to be more "mindful" of. Go to the dollar store and load up on stickers. (Toss some stickers and cheers into your suitcase too.) Then, start putting stickers on your chart—and celebrate when you do.

> Exactly what does that word mindful mean? Glad you asked – in the Leslie dictionary of life – it means 'stuff I want to pay attention to and notice'.

Will you feel silly? Maybe. But in the long run, who cares? You are taking care of yourself. You are not parking your car. You are making new ruts down that muddy road.

Now that you understand your brain wants to be happy, you can start setting some goals and deciding what your reward will be when you reach the goal. Keep in mind the principle of meeting you where you are.

I know you have this far-in-the-distance goal of reaching a certain weight, but we are not going to focus on that right now. I want you to see what is possible, and so many times, that goal weight feels impossible. Even though as Audrey Hepburn says, "Nothing is impossible, even the word says I'm possible." We don't want to set off the fear of failing, which triggers shaming and blaming. We have worked *too* hard to go down *that* road again.

Each week, I write down my goal in the same place where I track my food. I usually write my goal down on Friday, so I know where I am driving to that week. My goal may be to lose half a pound, walk 10,000 steps at least twice during the week, or not add cream to my coffee. You get the idea. (Notice not every goal is about losing weight.)

I also write down my reward next to my weekly goal. I like to make the reward match the effort. I may cheer for myself all the way home because I made great choices at the fast-food drive-thru all week. Other rewards have been a coffee from Starbucks, an extra-long visit with a friend, lipstick, and a new workout shirt. I rewarded myself with a Fitbit when I reached a major milestone (earlier I mentioned we would talk about the fitness watch? This is how I got mine!).

Mind Games, all about the games

Here is where mind games come into play. Let's pretend you set a goal to walk 5,000 steps three times a week and you decide your reward will be a fun pair of socks. But the weather is not great that week. You start thinking you "can't" get outside and walk.

Switch from thinking about the yucky weather to thinking about how much the fun pair of socks will make you smile. Then, put on your raincoat and rubber boots, set the timer on your phone for about five minutes (so you can turn around and walk back in about the same amount of time), and go walk. Once you get moving, add another two minutes to your timer. Imagine the socks, listen to your tunes, or use this time to listen to some great podcasts. Switching your focus from the yucky weather to how much you will enjoy the fun socks makes your brain happy and the walking more fun and less work. Yes, I know there are days when even the ducks stay home. On those days, I turn up the music and walk around in my house. The four-legged children have come to accept I am nuts; they usually ignore me. 😊

Start focusing on the rewards, not the goals. The goals usually involve denying ourselves something, and that is not fun. The rewards make our brains happy. The rewards make getting to the goal not feel like denial or work. (This feeds into your ***WHY.***) Thinking about rewards keeps us driving down the muddy road making new ruts. Driving down the muddy road gets us closer and closer to our destination.

What if you don't make it to your goal one week? Keep the same goal for the next week. Reflect on the reason you set that goal. (You can write the reason in your workbook too.) Refocus on the reward.

This is a journey. Remember the last trip you took? Did you change your destination just because you ran into traffic or faced a delay in boarding the plane? No. Same thing here. Do not park your car, do not get out, and do not walk home. Give yourself a cheer. You are still moving forward. You simply have not arrived, ***yet***. Yet is a very powerful word. Keep it close by.

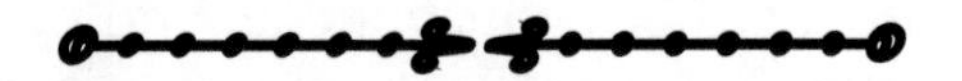

What's in your suitcase?

- Star stickers
- Fun stickers
- Fanny pack or phone holder if you don't have cordless headphones
- Gym membership
- Date for Free Session
- Quality workout shoes
- Rubber boots
- Raincoat
- Exercises for beginners
- Health app or fitness tracker
- Timer (a lot of phones have a timer)
- Alarm set to remind to go out and walk
- Headphones/music or podcasts
- Bigger megaphone
- Menu plan
- Grocery list
- More trash bags
- Hug from me
- Food plan/app
- Tracker – Fit and Food Journal
- Refillable oil sprayers for olive oil and regular oil (I prefer *Misto* brand)
- Food storage containers (my personal preference is the

Rubbermaid Freshworks Produce Saver – they work. Initial expense but you recover that in saved produce costs)
- More tissues
- Magnifying glass and binoculars to help spot triggers
- Choice – great choice, good choice, not so great choice
- Megaphone (for louder cheering!)
- Tissues
- Full-length photo
- Album set up in your phone or on your computer where you will store your "becoming you" photos
- No Should Zone t-shirt and poster
- Your power
- Google maps
- Locks
- "Traffic Jam" written on an index card
- Print off the "Stay" card
- Book of positive affirmations
- Seasoning
- Forgiveness
- Choices
- Community
- Stop
- Idea about your destination
- Plan for saboteurs
- Plan for food pushers
- Trash bags
- Oxygen mask
- ***WHY***
- Friedrich Nietzsche quote
- Photo of you
- Index cards
- Stake
- Hammer
- website
- Snap a photo – post it to the You Can't Eat Love Facebook page
- Join the private You Can't Eat Love Facebook group

- Workbook
- *So, I said to myself...*Journal
- Pens
- Highlighters

Life Hacks

- Buy some poster board or just get a piece of paper and create a chart of behaviors you want to change – each day you are successful – put up a sticker and do a happy dance! It's all about driving down that muddy road and making new ruts.
- Set goals each week AND decide on how you are going to reward yourself when you accomplish the goal. Set yourself up for success.
- If you don't reach your goal that week, keep the same goal and the same reward and refocus on the reward. You will get there!
- If a goal seems too big or too unreachable – break it down. I call it swiss cheesing something. Take one bite at a time, eventually, it will all be gone.

Jackie says

- Focus on perfect form and posture
- Don't be afraid to ask questions or to ask for help

Weblinks

https://linktr.ee/youcanteatlove

CHAPTER 16

Eeny, Meeny, Miney, Moe

“The secret of change is to focus all of your energy not on fighting the old, but on building the new.”

Socrates

Notice when you make good and great choices and cheer for yourself each time you make one of these choices. Then, notice how much easier it is to repeat the behavior the next time. This is the whole ***Don’t Shoot the Dog*** thing. We reward what we want the dog to do and ignore or redirect what we want the dog to stop doing. The same principle applies to you.

So, let's practice. Yes, practice. This is how you get the tires moving down a new patch of a very muddy road.

Pretend you bought two bags of chips for a party you are having later in the week. After doing a bit of housework, you feel snacky, and as my very dear friend Winnie the Pooh likes to say, you need a bit of a “smackerel.” (Of course, you don’t want to think about the “smackerel” too much, because you are hungry.) You open the cabinet, and there front and center, are the chips.

You decide you will have just a handful of chips. So, being mindful, you sit down at the table. (Pat yourself on the back for making a great choice to sit down at the table!) You open the bag, portion out a handful of chips (give yourself another pat), and savor them.

Then, you start looking at Facebook and Instagram on your phone. Your hand takes on a mind of its own. Suddenly, you realize you need to change the laundry. You look at the bag of chips and see it is empty.

> *I know you feel the shame trying to sneak in. Stop right there. No shame and blame are allowed here. Do not focus on what you did. Beating yourself up about it is not helpful.*

Think about what you will do differently next time. (Maybe you will put the bag back in the cabinet after you portion out the chips.) Throw away the empty bag. Forgive yourself.

Maybe even give yourself a bit of empathy. You could tell yourself, "I can only imagine how snacky you were. You have been working hard. Next time, let's..."

Empathy is different from sympathy. Empathy is having walked close to the other person's shoes so you draw from your own experience to gain an understanding of how they might be feeling. Sympathy is sharing in how the other person is feeling even though you might never have had that experience before.

In my humble opinion, having empathy for ourselves is very important. I discovered gaining an understanding of my emotions and why I felt the way I did enabled me to move past the not-so-great choices. After all, a lot of times, all I want is to be heard and seen, even if it is just by "myself." How about you?

What I hope you understand is to celebrate the wins, big or small, and ignore—absolutely, totally, completely ignore—anything else. Ignoring the things that are *not* wins dumps a little more dirt in the ruts, helping to slowly fill in the ruts.

If you think this sounds like baloney, just trust me. Try celebrating your wins for one week and note how your thinking is changing.

What we put into our brain is what comes out. To use a computer adage: garbage in, garbage out. Our brain is the most powerful computer in existence.

We also need to view our food as a source of fuel. What we take in affects what comes out of us too (e.g., our feelings, behaviors, etc.). Which fuel will you choose?

This journey will last the rest of your life. And you must determine what will and will not fit into your lifestyle. Remember you have choices—great, good, and not-so-good choices. (No bad choices here.)

If everyone keeps suggesting you eat non-fat Greek yogurt and the texture makes you gag, *it is ok to not eat it*. Do not waste your time (or calories) on things you do not like. *Enjoy* what you are eating.

Remember, quality food tastes so much better and satisfies more than quantities of food. That is why I now buy fresh fruits and vegetables and real butter and real mayonnaise. I am trading convenience for quality and flavor. I am worth the higher cost and the extra time it now takes to prepare my food.

I have finally come to understand my life, my money, and my time are my most valuable assets. If I do not treat them as cherished treasures, no one else will either. I am living my best life—and that is the best gift I can give me.

Are you ready to live your best life?

Feelings, again?

I want to take just a moment again to talk honestly with you about feelings. This is the hard part. This is also why your oxygen mask is so important.

So many times, we try to use our feelings to justify our not-so-good choices. I would say things like, “Because so and so made me feel such and such, I started eating everything that was not nailed down. If so and so did not... (fill in the blank), my life would be easier.”

But every time I said so and so made me... (fill in the blank), I actually was giving power to that person or event. By not taking responsibility for my choices, I was giving away a piece of myself—my power. I was saying I did not have power or control over parts of my life. I was helpless. I was admitting I have a terrible problem with food but saying it was not my fault.

No one in the world has the power to make you do anything you do not want to do. This includes being happy or mad. No one in this entire world has the power to *make you feel anything*. You have all the power in the world, and no one can take it away.

Starting today, notice when you say, “So and so made me...” Stop yourself. Think about what you are saying—and change your words.

I used to say certain people made me mad or sad. Now I say I feel mad or sad because of what certain people did. My new words focus on the behavior and not the person. Changing this thought process puts me in control and gives me back any power they may have been trying to steal from me (or that I was unknowingly giving away).

Then I will sit with the feeling until it passes. Just between us, if the feeling keeps growing and I am being pulled to the pantry or fridge, I will grab a protein drink, usually 1st Phorm Chocolate Milkshake. I mix eight ounces of cold water with one scoop of powder and shake it a few times. I feel less overwhelmed after drinking this. The creaminess reminds me of a milkshake. The chocolate flavor is usually what I am hunting for, and the protein helps calm my cravings. Remember, I am not a physician, dietician, or nutritionist. I am only sharing what works for me.

> Feelings are tough. Your workbook has a small section on feelings. The journal will give you more space to write. Oh, and by the way – no one can make you anything, except reservations for dinner!

Feelings will not hurt us. Not acknowledging and not looking at them will. Keep your power; **don't** give it away to anyone. Oxygen mask.

When the feeling has calmed down, I want you to give yourself a big cheer and a big hug and tell yourself how proud you are. High ten! I am proud of you too. You listened to how you were feeling, and you did not run from it. Celebrate! Make a note in your workbook of what you did to take care of yourself so you can remember what to do in the future.

Buy yourself a card

Do you like getting cards and letters in the mail? I do.

When I was in college, I would write letters to my mother. In one of the letters, I accused her of shipping me off and forgetting about me, because I had not heard from her in a while. Now, looking back, I understand my mother was overwhelmed with everything that was going on. My parents had just moved to Alaska, but that is a story for another day.

A couple of weeks after I sent the letter to my mother, she sent me a Hallmark Halloween card and a Hallmark Halloween pin in the mail. I still have them, and I still remember how I felt when I opened the card. Every Hallmark holiday from then until I graduated, my mother would send a card and a pin. I would wear the pins for thirty days before the holiday and feel her love each time I put them on.

I am telling you this story because cards may make a difference on your journey. They certainly made a difference on mine, especially when I started feeling a bit forgotten as I got further along on my journey.

One day, I was at the grocery store and happened to go down the card aisle. I noticed a card, stopped, and read it. I thought about how much I would enjoy receiving that card. Right then, I decided to buy the card for me.

When I got home, I wrote a note to myself in the card. I wrote the note to me from my very best friend in the whole wide world. I told myself how amazing I was and how proud I was of myself. I poured out as much love in that short space as I could. Then, I put the card into the envelope, sealed it, wrote my name on the outside, and put it with my food tracker.

The next time I felt like the journey was not worth it and like I wanted to park my car, I opened the card. I read it to myself. I cannot describe how I felt. I still reread that card and the many others I have added to the collection.

The next time you are at the store, look at the cards. Find one to send to your very best friend in the whole wide world. After you get home, sit down in a quiet place with your favorite pen and write that note to your very best friend in the whole wide world. Pour out your heart about how amazing they are and how proud you are of them.

Then, put the card into the envelope, seal the envelope, write your name on the outside of the envelope, and put the card where you will see it often. Take the card out and read it when you need to feel the encouragement and love that only a very best friend in the whole wide world can give. As the years go by, be sure to add to your collection. I would love to hear your stories about cards from *your* very best friend in the whole wide world.

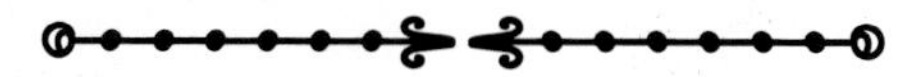

What's in your suitcase?

- Plan for after you make a not so great choice
- Protein Powder/Drink (my favorite is 1st Phorm Chocolate Milkshake)
- Greeting Cards
- Star stickers
- Fun stickers
- Fanny pack or phone holder if you don't have cordless headphones
- Gym membership
- Date for Free Session
- Quality workout shoes
- Rubber boots
- Raincoat
- Exercises for beginners
- Health app or fitness tracker
- Timer (a lot of phones have a timer)
- Alarm set to remind to go out and walk
- Headphones/music or podcasts
- Bigger megaphone

- Menu plan
- Grocery list
- More trash bags
- Hug from me
- Food plan/app
- Tracker – Fit and Food Journal
- Refillable oil sprayers for olive oil and regular oil (I prefer *Misto* brand)
- Food storage containers (my personal preference is the *Rubbermaid Freshworks Produce Saver* – they work. Initial expense but you recover that in saved produce costs)
- More tissues
- Magnifying glass and binoculars to help spot triggers
- Choice – great choice, good choice, not so great choice
- Megaphone (for louder cheering!)
- Tissues
- Full-length photo
- Album set up in your phone or on your computer where you will store your "becoming you" photos
- No Should Zone t-shirt and poster
- Your power
- Google maps
- Locks
- "Traffic Jam" written on an index card
- Print off the "Stay" card
- Book of positive affirmations
- Seasoning
- Forgiveness
- Choices
- Community
- Stop
- Idea about your destination
- Plan for saboteurs
- Plan for food pushers
- Trash bags
- Oxygen mask
- ***WHY***

- Friedrich Nietzsche quote
- Photo of you
- Index cards
- Stake
- Hammer
- website
- Snap a photo – post it to the You Can't Eat Love Facebook page
- Join the private You Can't Eat Love Facebook group
- Workbook
- *So, I said to myself...*Journal
- Pens
- Highlighters

Life Hacks

- Feelings. This was the hardest part of my journey. Becoming unafraid to face my real feelings and learning how to safely express myself. Sorting out the pieces and parts of anger. So many times, I was told not to feel, or I couldn't feel, or even worse, I shouldn't feel and I believed those people. Now, I know as a healthy human I MUST feel, or I am not able to live my very best life. If this is hard for you, just reach out, I will listen.

- Celebrating the things we want to continue helps deepen the ruts in our brains
- No one can make you anything. Don't give away your power
- Focus on behavior and not the person (including yourself)
- Letters/cards from your BFF help encourage you on the journey

Jackie says

- A good trainer is passionate
- A good trainer is relatable

Weblinks

https://linktr.ee/youcanteatlove

CHAPTER 17

Progress Not Perfection

It's a slow process, but quitting won't speed it up.

Anonymous

One of my favorite (and on some days, least favorite) expressions is "Rome was not built in a day." (This expression is attributed to John Heywood and the first recorded use of it was in 12th century Flanders, which we know as Belgium. Just a little interesting history.)

I tend to use this expression when someone is complaining about not completing a large task. I say it to remind them to look at their progress and see how far they *have* come, not so much how far they have to go.

Like you, I can get tangled up and frustrated with not arriving at a goal when I think I "should" or even when someone else thinks I "should." (There is that word we need to be sure to keep out of our vocabulary.) When I do, the shaming cycle starts, and I find myself driving my car down those old, familiar ruts in the muddy road.

Alcoholics Anonymous uses another expression that I like: "Progress not perfection." (You can use Google to find the entire expression, which is pretty powerful.) As you continue to make changes in your thinking and choices, you will begin to see progress, even if it is just a little bit.

Remember, you are driving your car down a very muddy road. You are trying to stay on the road and make new ruts. You do not drive ninety miles an hour; you creep along. You may not even have your foot on the gas, but you are moving forward, not backward. You *are* making progress.

The "not perfection" part of the expression is also true for this journey. We are not expecting ourselves to be perfect. We are learning to forgive ourselves and ignore the behaviors we *don't* want to continue. We are learning to acknowledge, celebrate, and reward the behaviors we *do* want to continue. Little by little, getting used to putting on our oxygen mask first, gaining control, and seeing tiny changes in ourselves.

I still remember when I had lost about twenty-five pounds. My weight loss was noticeable. I felt so proud of the work I was doing.

Around that time, I saw a friend I had not seen in a while. She commented on how good I looked. (I still wonder what she thought I looked like before.) She also said I should (yes, that word ☹) not lose any more weight. because I was going to be all wrinkly.

I smiled, thanked my friend for the "compliment," and then told myself, "I'm not that concerned about wrinkles. I only want to be the best me I can be."

When I went back to my *why* I noticed wrinkles did not have any role in my *why* or on my journey. They were going to be what they were going to be. I did what I could by buying a higher quality moisturizer (although I am not certain that has made any difference) and then chose to not worry about wrinkles.

I understand not wanting to have excess skin hanging off you. I was genuinely concerned about having a double chin and saggy arms. This was part of what inspired me to work out.

When we work out, we strengthen, tighten, and tone our muscles. Since our skin lies on top of our muscles, we usually see some tightening of the skin too. How much depends on your age and how much weight you lose.

But much like a stretched-out pair of socks, all of our body may not be able to be like "new." I have accepted that. I still wear cute, sleeveless tops. Be bold. You have worked hard.

Paper or Google Maps?

Just like on a real trip, we need to see how far we have come. On the airplane, I love to look at the flight path map. The line behind the plane is solid while the line in front of the plane is dotted and can change depending on the weather and things like that. On this journey, we have several mile markers we can look at to see how far we have traveled.

At the start of my journey, I decided I would get rid of my clothes when they got too loose. I would do this regardless of what item it was, how much I loved it, or the memories it stirred up. (Ok, I kept the pants I wore the first time I officially weighed myself when I began this journey. That is the *only* item of clothing I kept.)

If I put an item of clothing on and it was loose, I would choose to either wear it and then wash it and get rid of it, or I would change my clothes and get rid of it right away. Most of the time, since I was already dressed, I chose to wear the item and then washed it and got rid of it.

I kept a bag in my closet so I could put items in the bag as soon as they came out of the wash. When the bag got about half full, I would take it to a local ministry. The loose clothes were gone. It was that easy. I got rid of probably 200 pounds of clothes on my journey—almost a two for one.

So, your assignment right now is to find a trash bag and at least one item that no longer fits or does not make you smile when you wear it. Put the item in the trash bag. Then, put the bag where it will be easy for you to drop in the clothes that are not going to fit anymore.

Each time you put your laundry away, I want you to look at your clothes and get rid of items that are loose or do not make you smile when you wear them. Yes, I can hear you talking about the expense and how you can have them taken in and all of that. But be honest with yourself. Do you really want to surround yourself with clothes that don't show off the best you that you are becoming? I didn't think so.

You are working so hard to change your thoughts. You are working so hard to discover who *you* are. And you are working so hard to learn to love yourself as much as you deserve to be loved. You deserve new clothes that fit you *now* where you are on your journey.

So, what did I do as I emptied my closet and my drawers? (Yes, even pitch your unmentionables as they become more mentionable.) I went shopping.

Now, I didn't go to any of the high-end retailers. I stuck to Walmart, Target, JCPenney, and Kohl's. (Both JCPenney and Kohl's have amazing sales). I didn't invest a lot of money in the clothes I bought during this stage of my journey, because I knew it was just a matter of time before the clothes went into the bag. (I did spend a wee bit more on unmentionables, just because.)

I learned a trick to meet my need for pants. I would buy pants that had belt loops and were made of stretchy fabric (not yoga pants). I would buy them just a smidge tight. I knew in about a month or two they would fit just right. (Size-wise, my rule of thumb is to go down a size for every ten pounds). So, my logic was that I could get three sizes out of one pair of pants—the smidge tight, the just right, and the slightly baggy. I only had about four pairs of pants that fit during this time.

When the pants hit the slightly baggy stage, their next stop was the bag, and I would get a new pair of pants. I did the same thing with tops and pajamas. My trick for staying in tops was to shop in the athletic wear section. The fabric had a bit of stretch to it and prices were a lot more reasonable. I could also choose from a good selection of colors.

Please do not hold onto baggy tops. Catching a glimpse of yourself in a baggy top can let a lot of air out of your balloon. You only want to wear things that make you smile when you see yourself. You are doing a lot of hard work. You need to celebrate when you see yourself.

> *I observed something on the journey that nobody talks about it. After I had lost about thirty pounds, I noticed I was cold more often. I have not done any research to figure out why. I just wear a jacket and put a blanket on my bed.*

I have a suggestion on how to keep your pants up as you change sizes. I discovered my best bet was to buy a belt that was woven and didn't have any holes in it. I put the buckle through the weave. This way, I didn't have to keep buying belts because the holes were not where I needed them to be. (Add a woven belt to your suitcase.)

Another belt trick I learned is to thread the belt one loop back from the front loop. This puts the buckle over my hip and not my stomach. I discovered the belt and my pants would lay more smoothly, and I liked how that looked. Try it and let me know what you think.

Paparazzi warning

Smile! This is a very important piece of your journey. I want you to take a photo of yourself on the same day of each month, so you can see how you are changing. Put the photo into a folder on your phone and your computer.

I realized when I looked at myself in a mirror, I would focus only on certain parts of myself. I would not allow myself to look at the parts I did not like or of which I was ashamed. But I could see ***all*** of myself at one time when I looked at a photo.

As the months passed, I could see the changes happening in my body. I am grateful I have those photo reminders of where I have been. And you will be too. You can print them out and put them in your workbook or just store them in an album on your phone and computer.

When you hit a traffic jam and you are tempted to get out and walk home, pull out your photos and see exactly how far you have come. On some of those bad traffic days, take a quick photo so you can get a quick visual of the work you have done.

Have you ever heard someone say they still see themselves as they used to be? Our brains are used to seeing things the way they have been recorded. That is how we recognize people and objects.

As we change, our brain must repaint the memory of what we look like. Photos can help with the repainting. Photos can help your brain see you as you are now and not as you were, and this is very important to your journey.

So, take photos. Look at them. Repaint *you* in *your* brain.

Stay in your car. No parking. No getting out. No walking home. Move forward, making new ruts on the muddy roads.

Bags of dog food

I know sometimes you might feel like this journey is just not worth it. Remember, we are breaking this down bit by bit. Progress, not perfection. We are not parking our car, getting out, and walking home.

On one of those days when you think "this" is not worth it, I want you to go to the grocery store or the pet supply store. You don't have to buy anything. Just go to the store and grab a cart on your way in.

Go to the dog food section. You know how much weight you have lost, right? Well, I want you to stack bags of dog food in your cart that equal how much weight you have lost. Look at the bags. Do you see how much it is?

Now, I want you to pick up all those bags and walk up and down the full length of the pet food aisle at least twice. I want you to feel the weight of those bags of dog food. Think about what you were asking your body, especially your knees and feet, to do for you.

After completing this little walk/exercise, you can put the bags down. I want you to feel how much lighter you are.

Soak in what you have accomplished. Do a happy dance right there in the aisle.
Then, get in your car and loudly cheer for yourself the entire way home. I am so very proud of what you have done. I would love to hear from you so we can celebrate together.

How did I come up with this crazy idea? Well, when I decided I had lost all the weight I believed I could keep off, I told Jackie. (Notice I did not say my goal or how much I lost, but how much I believed I could keep off, the weight at which I was certain I could live.)

At the end of my workout, Jackie and I went to the rack with the super heavy dumbbells. She told me to pick up two forty-eight-and-a-half-pound dumbbells and walk from one end of the gym to the other end of the gym without stopping. Yikes! I had asked my back, my knees, and my feet to carry that much extra weight daily.

I will never forget that "exercise" in the gym. I had a total understanding of the demand I had put on my body. I could have sat down and cried if I had not been so excited when I finally grasped what I had done.

So, carry the dog food. You will be glad you did.

I have done something else to remind myself of how much weight I am no longer carrying. I have donated flour, sugar, and canned goods that add up to the amount of weight I have lost. This can be a very impactful visual—and food pantries always need food. (Share on our Facebook page. Who knows who you might inspire!)

What's in your suitcase?

- Progress not perfection
- Bag/Trash bag for clothes that don't fit
- Woven belt
- Photo taken about the same date each month – put in a folder on your phone or computer
- Dog food 😊
- Happy Dance music!!
- Plan for after you make a not so great choice
- Protein Powder/Drink (my favorite is 1st Phorm Chocolate Milkshake)
- Greeting Cards
- Star stickers
- Fun stickers
- Fanny pack or phone holder if you don't have cordless headphones
- Gym membership
- Date for Free Session
- Quality workout shoes
- Rubber boots
- Raincoat
- Exercises for beginners
- Health app or fitness tracker
- Timer (a lot of phones have a timer)
- Alarm set to remind to go out and walk
- Headphones/music or podcasts
- Bigger megaphone
- Menu plan
- Grocery list
- More trash bags
- Hug from me
- Food plan/app
- Tracker – Fit and Food Journal
- Refillable oil sprayers for olive

oil and regular oil (I prefer *Misto* brand)

- Food storage containers (my personal preference is the *Rubbermaid Freshworks Produce Saver* – they work. Initial expense but you recover that in saved produce costs)
- More tissues
- Magnifying glass and binoculars to help spot triggers
- Choice – great choice, good choice, not so great choice
- Megaphone (for louder cheering!)
- Tissues
- Full-length photo
- Album set up in your phone or on your computer where you will store your "becoming you" photos
- No Should Zone t-shirt and poster
- Your power
- Google maps
- Locks
- "Traffic Jam" written on an index card
- Print off the "Stay" card
- Book of positive affirmations
- Seasoning
- Forgiveness
- Choices
- Community
- Stop
- Idea about your destination
- Plan for saboteurs
- Plan for food pushers
- Trash bags
- Oxygen mask
- ***WHY***
- Friedrich Nietzsche quote
- Photo of you
- Index cards
- Stake
- Hammer
- website
- Snap a photo – post it to the You

Can't Eat Love Facebook page
- Join the private You Can't Eat Love Facebook group
- Workbook
- *So, I said to myself...*Journal
- Pens
- Highlighters

Life Hacks

- If the journey is feeling overwhelming, look back at how far you have come. Look over your tracker and see the positive changes you have been making. Look at your photos and enjoy seeing you being revealed.
- Don't keep any clothes that either don't fit or that you don't feel amazing in when you put them on
- Buckle your belt to the side
- Taking a photo about the same date each month helps our brains repaint how it sees us. Don't be afraid to take more than one a month. It will help your brain realize a new you is here and the old you is gone.

Jackie says

- A good trainer walks the walk

Weblinks

https://linktr.ee/youcanteatlove

CHAPTER 18

You Do Not Have To Do This Alone

"Alone we can do so little; together we can do so much."
Helen Keller

We have talked about a lot. One thing I hope you have learned as we have traveled on this journey is how powerful your mind is. Recently, I heard a quote that summed up all this "car driving down a muddy road' stuff for me.

In ***Man's Search for Meaning***, Viktor Frankl said, "Between stimulus and response there is a space. In that space is our power to choose our response. In our response lies our growth and our freedom." (Frankl, 2006)

Let's think about that for a moment. When something happens like a meal is served or a snack is suggested, we can take a moment. We can take a breath, pause, think, and choose. We have the power to choose how we respond, and we can be kind and loving to ourselves. If we take that moment, that breath, that pause and decide to make certain our response lines up with our ***WHY***, we will never doubt our actions.

Take control. Have power. Be free. How amazing is that?

I am responsible for my feelings. I will not give my power away, because I want to be in control of my response. I want to grow and be free.

Are there people in your life who will not like the "new you"? Yes, there are. Why? Because you have chosen you first. You have decided you are worth putting on your own oxygen mask first before you help anyone else. And you are growing into the real you. People do not like change. Especially the people who are close to us who are *not* changing.

We return to not shooting the dog. We have taught the people in our life how to treat us. Now, we are teaching them to treat us differently. Yes, old dogs can be taught new tricks.

I want you to understand you are not alone. Reach out to me if you need to. I will listen.

The information, ideas, and discussions I have shared with you did not just appear in my mind. Yes, I do have quite a few crazy thoughts, but on occasion, someone else's thoughts sent me down the path or validated my thoughts. I will share some of these resources with you so you can check them out yourself.

Through Adult Children of Alcoholics and Dysfunctional Families, I came to understand I am only responsible for *my* feelings. I learned what feelings are and how to look at them even though I was terrified. By learning about my feelings, my protective armor started cracking and I realized there was a possibility I was lovable. Imperfect, but lovable. Not only that, I *deserve* to be loved. This was a concept that took me a bit of time to accept.

I still remember trying to do an exercise where I would look in the mirror every morning at a certain time. The exercise was to look straight into my eyes and repeat three times, "I love you." I could not do it. Tears would fill my eyes. I could not look right at my own eyes and tell myself I loved me. I felt broken.

As I continued the work of learning about my feelings, the exercise got a bit easier. Now, I can look at my beautiful, very blue eyes and tell myself, "I love you." Tears fill my eyes for a different reason now. They fill my eyes because I feel the love going between us.

I also started reading Proverbs in the Bible. There are thirty-one proverbs, which very nicely works out to one a day in each month. I read what I call the Proverb of the Day. For example, on the first of the month, I read Proverb 1. Pretty simple. I am not telling you to read or not read the Bible. I am just letting you know the things I did to learn to love myself. At first, when I would read the Proverbs, I felt as if it were a waste of time, but then I started seeing affirmations of what a good person I was. Reading those affirmations daily helped me start my day off in a positive direction.

I would suggest browsing a Hallmark store (or the Hallmark website) or a bookstore (if there is one close by) for a book with affirmations or entries that bring a smile to your face when you read them. Buy a book like this for yourself. Again, you deserve it.

I have the book, ***Now is the Time to...***, from Hallmark. I have read it almost every morning for the past five years. I make notes to myself and date them so I can reflect on the comments when I read them again several months or years later.

Another book of affirmations I would recommend is ***ANEW Spiritual Awakening: 31-Day Christian Devotional, Let God's Love Transform Life's Brokenness Into Something Beautiful*** by JV Lauren. There is a workbook that goes along with the book. Remember, garbage in, garbage out. Start filling your brain with quality goodness. *You* are worth it.

I also read ***Getting the Love You Want*** by Harville Hendrix. On this journey, I learned the most important relationship in my life is the one I have with myself. To thrive, I had to learn to love myself. I needed some direction with that, and this book provided that direction. It also helped me with my other relationships. (Oxygen mask. *Don't shoot the dog*.)

I mentioned before that I followed the Weight Watchers program. Weight Watchers taught me what to eat and how much to eat for a balanced diet. The word diet is appropriate here because it refers to food.

The Beck Diet Solution by Judith S. Beck also provided a scientific background for the work I was doing to change my thought process. She applies Cognitive Behavior Therapy (CBT) to weight loss. (CBT focuses on modifying dysfunctional emotions, behaviors, and thoughts by questioning irrational thoughts and beliefs. It is considered a "solutions-oriented" form of talk therapy.) The book covers forty-two days of guided practice to help change your thoughts and beliefs about food. There is also an audiobook. (Beck 2007)

If you are looking for an easy-to-read and understand guide to nutrition and calories, I suggest ***The Weight Loss Code: A Practical Guide to Sustainable Weight*** by Yemi Fadipe. It is also available as an e-book. The author does a great job of breaking down the "What" and "How" behind calories and nutrition.

By now, you are learning a lot of new skills and working on your new habits. One of my favorite books about thinking differently is ***The Magic of Thinking Big*** by David J Schwartz. Yes, it is a book written about businesses and for businesspeople. Consider this. Aren't you the CEO of the most important company in the world—you? So, a lot of these principles apply. A couple of my favorites are thinking three positive thoughts each night before you go to sleep and having a Big Hairy Audacious Goal or BHAG for short.

Remember our brain likes to be happy, and it is incredibly good at making up stories. If the last thoughts we have before falling asleep are pleasant, that will make our brain happy. And we can go back to the garbage thing. Filling our brains with pleasant thoughts helps us to keep making new ruts on the muddy road.

I am going to take a few liberties with his BHAG philosophy. To create lasting change in ourselves, I believe we need to have a Big Hairy Audacious Why or BHAW (not to be confused with the TV show Hee Haw or the playground toy see-saw). You already see your ***WHY*** is what is going to keep you in the car and moving forward.

So, dig down deep and find your "this is my life's dream" ***WHY***. Write it down, copy it, and put it where you see it all the time. When the journey gets tough, you know what to do. Get out your ***WHY***, remember, and keep moving forward. Progress, not perfection.

Learning to love myself was difficult. So much of my life was spent making everyone else happy. Losing myself was the cost. Food was definitely my drug of choice, and I insulated myself in the results.

Someone kept recommending I read ***Self-Compassion*** by Kristin Neff, Ph.D., and I kept ignoring the comment. Finally, I broke down and bought the book only to leave

it sitting on the shelf. Maybe I was expecting to read it by osmosis. I don't know.
I started learning more and more about myself. I started being kinder to myself. I started learning what I did not know. I stumbled across ***Self-Compassion*** on the shelf where it had been sitting for some time. I started reading it and could not put it down. I felt as if it was the missing piece to the puzzle. I want to share a couple of the quotes that helped me know I was on the right path. I simply needed more information.

> *"We look in the mirror and don't like what we see (both literally and figuratively), and the shame starts to set in."*
>
> *"Self-criticism—despite being socially sanctioned—was not at all helpful, and in fact only made things worse. I wasn't making myself a better person by beating myself up all the time... I wasn't owning up to many things because I was so afraid of the self-hate that would follow if I admitted the truth."*

I would encourage you to add the book, ***Self-Compassion***, to your suitcase. The author does a great job tackling that hard subject of shame. The book includes helpful, guided exercises so you can practice self-compassion. My copy is underlined, highlighted, and tabbed. Make sure you have pens and highlighters when you sit down to read. I am certain you will want to mark the parts that speak to you. (Neff, 2011)

I would also suggest you check out two books by Harriet Lerner, Ph.D. – ***The Dance of Anger*** and ***The Dance of Connection***. The ***Dance of Anger*** can help you dig down under that feeling and begin to see what is driving it, more importantly, you will learn some skills to manage it. ***The Dance of Connection*** can help you learn how to speak to other people, so you feel heard, get out of the middle of conversations you don't belong in, and build better relationships with the important people in your life.

Three other books you might want to add to your reading list are ***Forgiveness is Power*** by William Fergus Martin (We need to learn how and why to forgive ourselves and others.), ***Boundaries*** by Dr. Henry Cloud and Dr. John Townsend (Part of the oxygen mask is knowing how to clearly define our boundaries.) and ***Oola, Find Balance in an Unbalanced World*** by Dave Braun and Troy Amdahl (You can explore the different areas of your life and see where you can get a better balance.).

One more resource I want to mention to you is ***Atomic Habits*** by James Clear. He breaks down how habits are formed, how to change them, and why it is so difficult to get rid of bad habits. He takes a little-by-little approach to change. Little motivations help you keep moving forward. (Clear, 2018)

You are on a journey to change your relationship with food, and a large part of that relationship is based on habit. ***Atomic Habits*** can give you the nuts, bolts, and framework to have the relationship you do want with food. His approach helps you drive your car down that very muddy road and make new ruts and reward the behavior you want to continue.

The last resource I want to suggest is ***The Miracle Morning*** by Hal Elrod. He helps you develop a "first thing in the morning" plan to set you up for success for the rest of your day. This is a simple approach to gaining control and taking charge of your life. This is one of the kindest things you can do for yourself. (Oxygen mask – I have started calling my morning time my "gardening time". I am tending to the most important plant/crop in my life – me) Please share how you are taking care of you first thing in the morning and more importantly, the impact it is having on the rest of your day.

My hope is you realize you are never alone. Between me and these resources, you have almost everything you need to stay in your car and keep moving forward on this journey.

So, I guess this is where I get out and you continue this journey. I am just an email, Facebook post, or private message away. I hope you have learned what an amazing person *I think* you are—because that is *how amazing you are*.

But, *before* we do a final inventory of everything in your suitcase, I want to leave you with a couple more quotes from Viktor Frankl from ***Man's Search for Meaning*** (Frankl, 2006):

> *"When we are no longer able to change a situation, we are challenged to change ourselves."*
>
> *"Those who have a 'why' to live, can bear with almost any 'how.'"*

You have your Big Hairy Audacious Why. Now go live ***your*** absolute best life.

Let's pull out your suitcase and take an inventory. I want to make certain you have everything you need.

What's in your suitcase?

- A breath, a moment, a pause
- Book of Affirmations or Inspirations
- BHAW (Big Hairy Amazing ***WHY***)
- *Self-Compassion* by Kristin Neff, PhD
- More pens and highlighters
- *Miracle Morning* – help get your day started with a great mindset
- Progress not perfection
- Bag/Trash bag for clothes that don't fit
- Woven belt
- Photo taken about the same date each month – put in a folder on your phone or computer
- Dog food 😊
- Happy Dance music!!
- Plan for after you make a not so great choice
- Protein Powder/Drink (my favorite is 1st Phorm Chocolate Milkshake)
- Greeting Cards
- Star stickers
- Fun stickers
- Fanny pack or phone holder if you don't have cordless headphones
- Gym membership
- Date for Free Session
- Quality workout shoes
- Rubber boots
- Raincoat
- Exercises for beginners
- Health app or fitness tracker
- Timer (a lot of phones have a timer)

- Alarm set to remind to go out and walk
- Headphones/music or podcasts
- Bigger megaphone
- Menu plan
- Grocery list
- More trash bags
- Hug from me
- Food plan/app
- Tracker – Fit and Food Journal
- Refillable oil sprayers for olive oil and regular oil (I prefer *Misto* brand)
- Food storage containers (my personal preference is the *Rubbermaid Freshworks Produce Saver* – they work. Initial expense but you recover that in saved produce costs)
- More tissues
- Magnifying glass and binoculars to help spot triggers
- Choice – great choice, good choice, not so great choice
- Megaphone (for louder cheering!)
- Tissues
- Full-length photo
- Album set up in your phone or on your computer where you will store your "becoming you" photos
- No Should Zone t-shirt and poster
- Your power
- Google maps
- Locks
- "Traffic Jam" written on an index card
- Print off the "Stay" card
- Book of positive affirmations
- Seasoning
- Forgiveness
- Choices
- Community
- Stop
- Idea about your destination

- Plan for saboteurs
- Plan for food pushers
- Trash bags
- Oxygen mask
- ***WHY***
- Friedrich Nietzsche quote
- Photo of you
- Index cards
- Stake
- Hammer
- website
- Snap a photo – post it to the You Can't Eat Love Facebook page
- Join the private You Can't Eat Love Facebook group
- Workbook
- *So, I said to myself...*Journal
- Pens
- Highlighters

Life Hacks

- I'm just curious...
- I hear you saying...
- Right now, I am working to be the best me I can be.

Jackie says

- A good trainer listens to what you are saying
- A good trainer inspires you

Weblinks

https://linktr.ee/youcanteatlove

Not the very end; just the beginning

The phone is ringing. (Caller ID – BFFITWWW)
"Hello?"
"Hello, this is you."
"You? I'm me!"
"I know. I am just calling to tell you I think you are one of the most amazing people I have ever met. I wanted to let you know when you are struggling, I believe in you. No matter what. You've got this. I want you to believe in you as much as I do."

"And one last thing. You don't need to try and fill that *myself*-sized hole in your heart. I have filled it for you."

"You no longer need to eat love. I love *you* just as *you are*."

You are enough.

Free online course on
Triggers, Choices, and Celebrations
https://youcanteatlove.com/free-course

If you have gotten as much from reading this book as I did from sharing it with you, please leave a review. Your review will help other people discover this book. https://www.bklnk.com/review/B08RYC6Y8F

With gratitude,
Leslie Lindsey Davis
December 2020

Acknowledgments

Gratitude turns what we have into enough.

Melody Beattie

Just like most things we do in life; we don't do it alone. None of us live in a vacuum. I want to thank so many people on my journey. I hope I don't miss anyone, but if I do, the fault is all mine and not deliberate.

Thank you to the Pfishin' Sisters, Kathy, Isa, and Allison. I treasure your encouragement, insight, laughs, reading, and suggestions. You are used to my crazy ideas and never hesitate to go along for the ride, even if only because you sometimes have crazier ideas. 😊

Thank you to my youngest son, Matthew. Several years back, you told me to go and do something amazing. Each time I step into a new adventure, I try and measure it against that stick and wonder if you will think what I'm doing is amazing enough.

Thank you to my second son, Jeffrey. The day Gabby (my tiny toy poodle) died, I told you I was sad. As you hugged me, you said, "Of course you're sad." You may never understand how much your words meant to me. Before learning to love myself, I would not have been able to say my words out loud.

Thank you to my oldest son, Philip. Despite everything, the gift you gave me was the push to find a better way, to examine the past, to determine to become the best version of myself—the version that loves me just as I am, and to fill the myself-sized hole in my heart. By filling the hole, I can unselfishly love you despite the separation.

Thank you to my husband, Mike. I can't wait to see what adventures are ahead.

I also want to say thank you to Donna, Eretha, Erika, Laura, Lorna, Michele, Valerie, and Verna. You were with me every step of the way on the weight loss part of my journey, and you are now some of my dearest friends. You always had a smile, a hug, and an encouraging word. You celebrated with me and picked me up when I felt like giving up. I counted on you to say exactly what I needed to hear each week. I cannot imagine taking this journey without you.

Thank you to all the people who sat in the room with me at the beginning, the middle, and the end of my weight loss journey. Thank you for celebrating with me. I will always be grateful for how patiently you listened to my crazy stories (many of which are here in this book).

Thank you to Jackie who met me where I was and believed I could do more. Your unwavering belief in me kept me coming back week after week. Little by little I got stronger, my body transformed, and I grew in confidence. Thank you for celebrating the little wins and the big wins. Thank you for never letting me give up on myself.

Thank you to Malinda who so graciously offered to read the manuscript of a stranger and now I count her as one of my friends. Your honest insight, gentle corrections, and inspirational suggestions helped me to deliver a more complete manuscript to the editor. I will be forever honored by your generosity.

Thank you to Michelle, my editor. As I tried to find the words to thank you, my eyes filled with tears. Your constant affirmation I was on the right track with what I was saying made my heart and spirit just soar. You took a ragged blanket and turned it into something amazing. You have such a gift to give my words life.

Thank you to Katie Chambers who so very kindly offered to help me when I struggled with the content on the back of the book. I was so grateful for your quick and kind offer to help.

Thank you to Chandler Bolt, Self-Publishing School. You kept the four-legged children and me company for hours on end as we walked the back of the property. I am so grateful for the offer of the Six-Day, Six-Figure Challenge. That Challenge gave me the courage to submit my first manuscript to an editor. Then I was challenged to believe I could write and publish this book in about 90 days. Chandler, books do change lives. Thank you for the push.

Thank you to Anthony, Self-Publishing School, who kept talking to me until I believed, with the help of Self-Publishing School, I could bring this book to life. That and a common weightlifting interest always makes the conversations interesting. Anthony, I will reach 225lbs and you will be the second person I tell.

Thank you to Ellaine who talked me through so many of my doubts. Your kindness and patience are incredible gifts. I was so grateful to say you were my coach. When I grow up, I hope I am just like you.

Thank you to Michael who provided the perfectly timed supply of the perfectly sized Diet Coke. I will never see another bottle of Diet Coke without remembering your kindness and thoughtfulness. I was able to finish.

Thank you to all the SPS family. It was so comforting to know we were all rowing different boats in the same water. I was so grateful for all the times you lifted me with just the right words.

Thank you to Scott who formatted this book and the workbook. You understood my message and put the perfect finish on the words. You are a true artist.

Finally, thank you to Micah and the team at 100 Covers. I sent you a few crazy ideas, the first few paragraphs of the work, and a title. What you returned was pure magic. I am so grateful you understood and were able to translate my vision into a stunning cover. Now, I pray my words are worthy of your masterpiece.

"When we are no longer able to change a situation, we are challenged to change ourselves."

Viktor Frankl

To schedule a call and talk about your next steps
https://youcanteatlove.com/contact-me

References

Webster Illustrated Contemporary Dictionary – Encyclopedic Edition. United States of America; JG Ferguson Publishing Company, 1988.

Lauren, JV. Anew Spiritual Awakening: 31 – Day Christian Devotional, Let God's Love Transform Life's Brokenness Into Something Beautiful. 2020.

Beck, Judith S. Ph.D. The Beck Diet Solution, Train Your Brain to Think Like a Thin Person. New York: Oxmoor House, 2007.

Pryor, Karen. Don't Shoot the Dog!: The New Art of Teaching and Training. Lydney: Ringpress Books, 2006.

Neff, Kristin, Ph.D. Self-Compassion: The Proven Power of Being Kind to Yourself. New York: William Morrow, 2011.

Clear, James. Atomic Habits: An Easy & Proven Way to Build Good Habits & Break Bad Ones. New York: Avery, 2018.

About the Author

Leslie Lindsey Davis is always on a journey. Her motto is "why not?". She measures things she wants to do against the yardstick of "When I am 80 years old, I don't want to be sitting in my rocking chair on my front porch saying, 'I wish I would have'".

She has taken a wrong turn on several trips with her older boys. The boys would say "we're lost". Her reply was always, "No, we are on an adventure."

Life is one grand adventurous journey and making sure everything is done from scuba diving to beekeeping. From riding on an elephant to riding in a hot air balloon. And so much more in between.

Her passions, besides her family, are GUTaS International and her heart family in Zimbabwe – especially Mercy, Betty, and Itai. GUTaS stands for Get Up, Take a Step. GUTaS is changing lives one step, one stitch at a time.

When her husband and children ask "Why?" Her response is always "Why not."

If we have our own why in life, we can get along with almost any how.

Friedrich Nietzsche

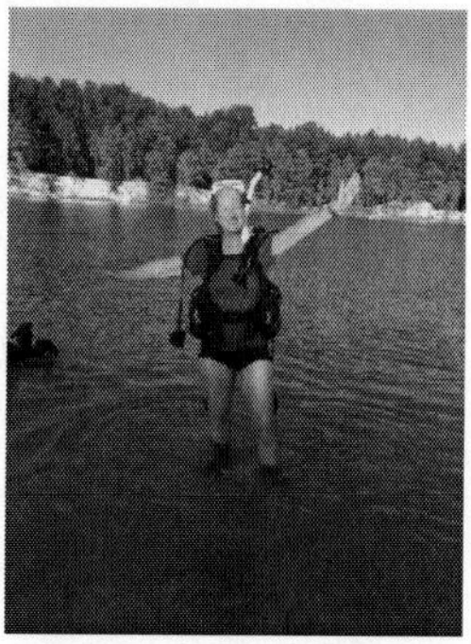

Made in United States
North Haven, CT
19 November 2023